Amyloidosis - History and Perspectives

Edited by Jonathan S. Harrison

Published in London, United Kingdom

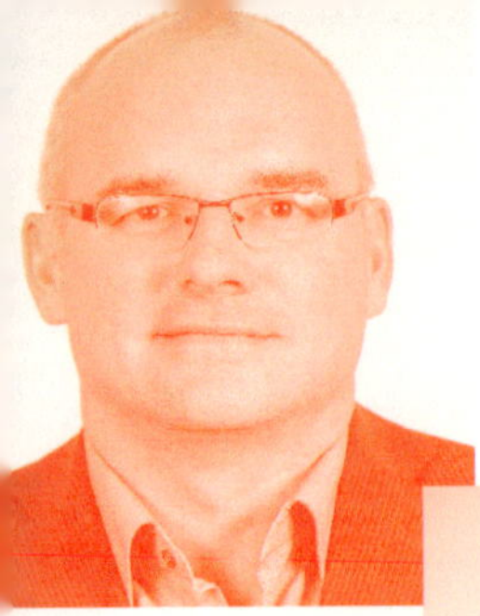
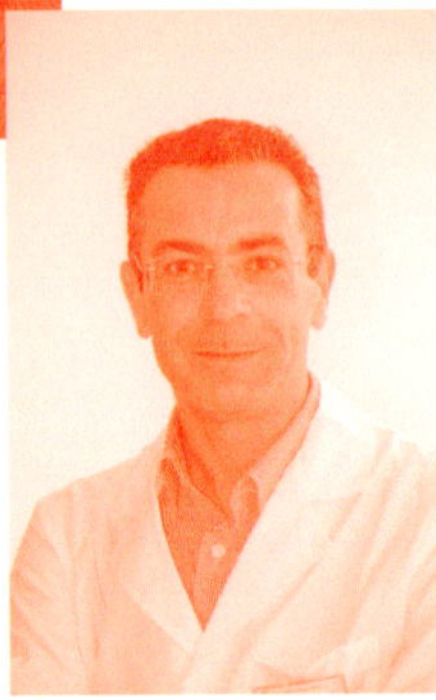
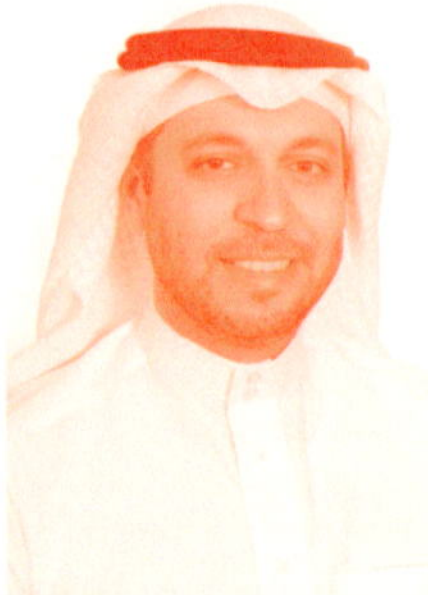
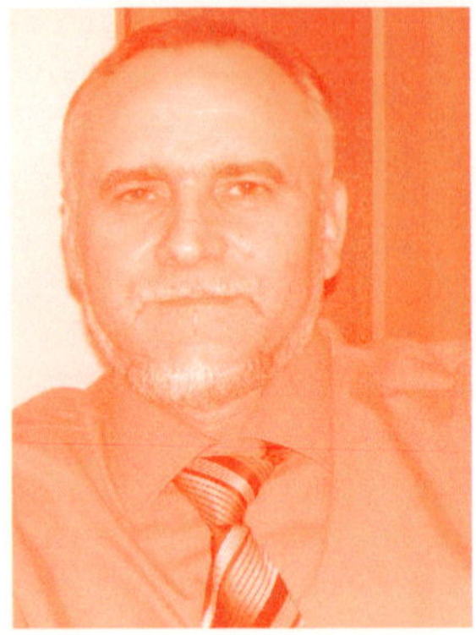
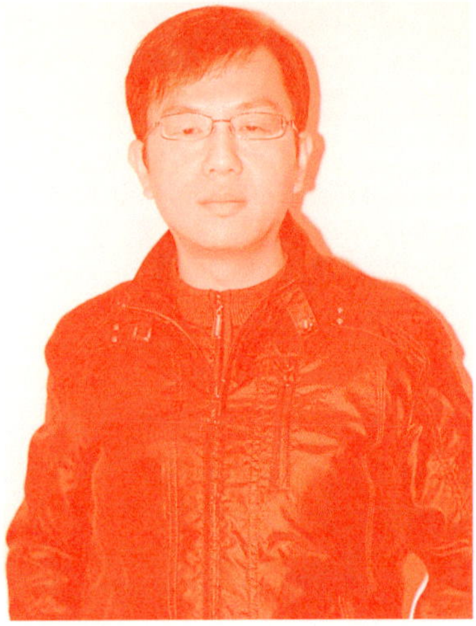
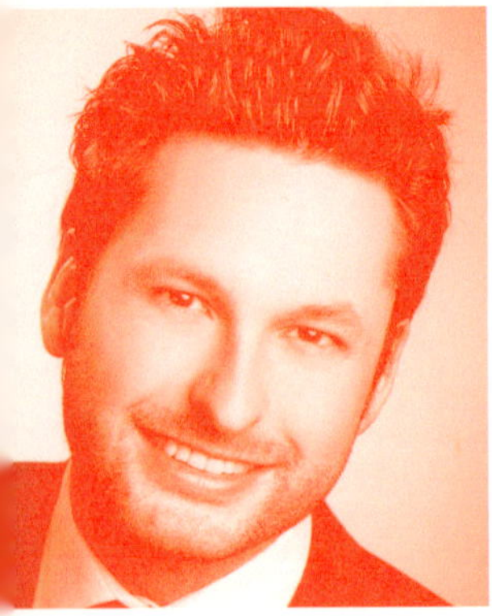
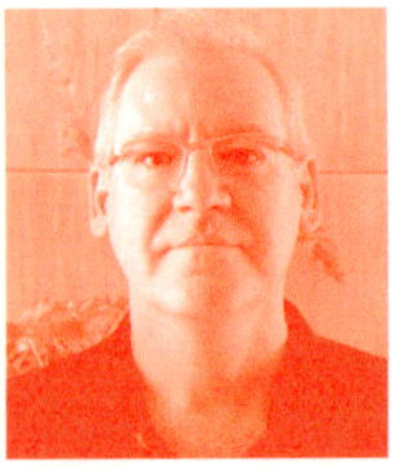

IntechOpen

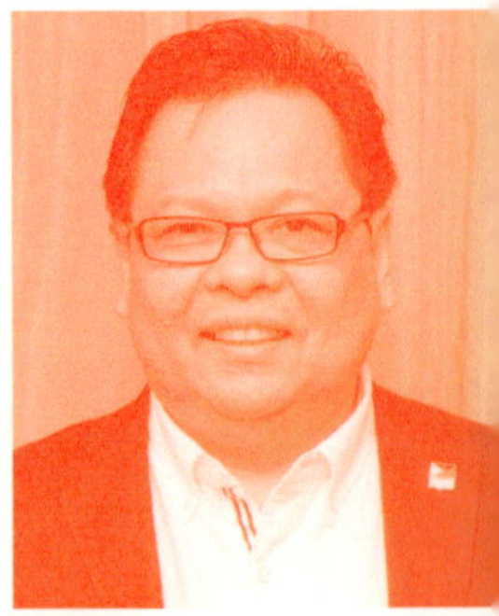
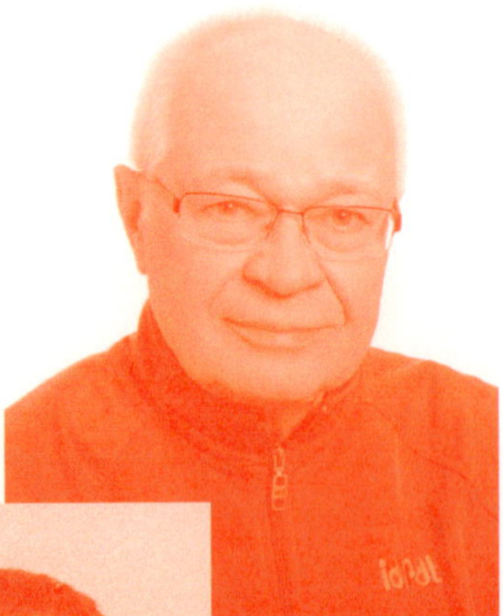
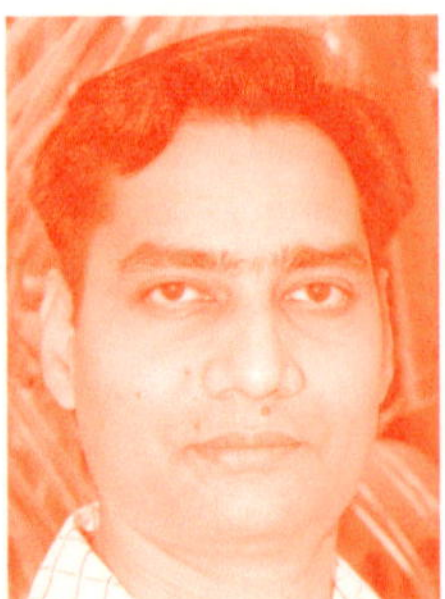
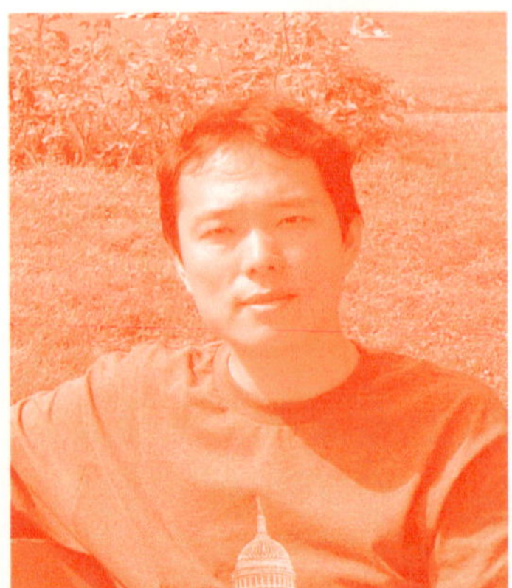
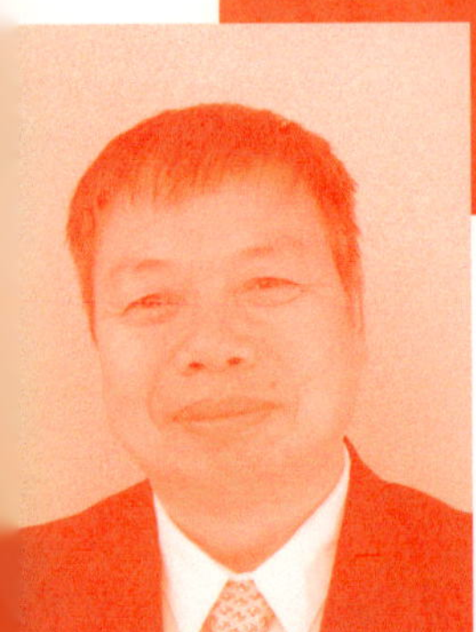
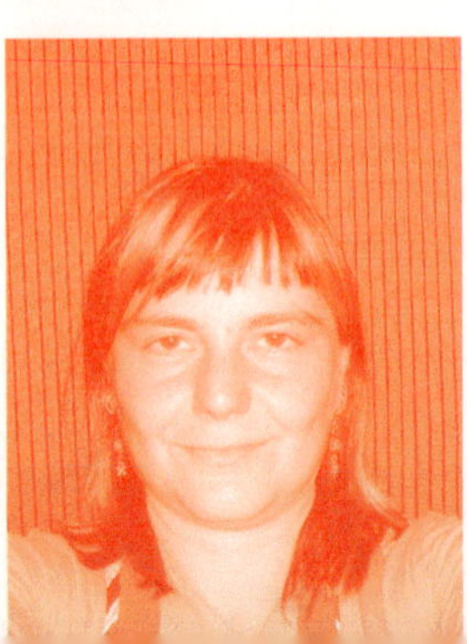

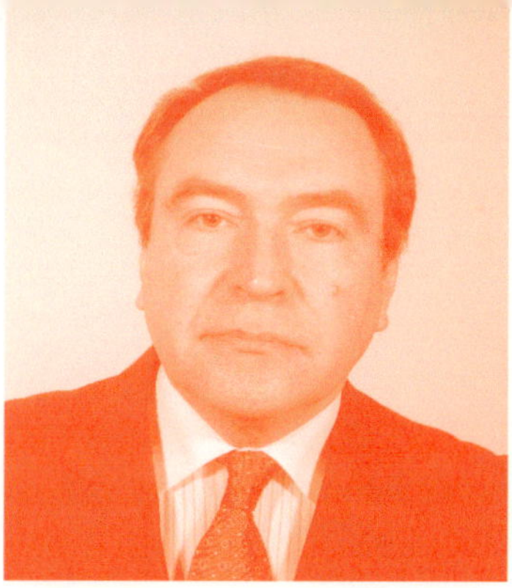

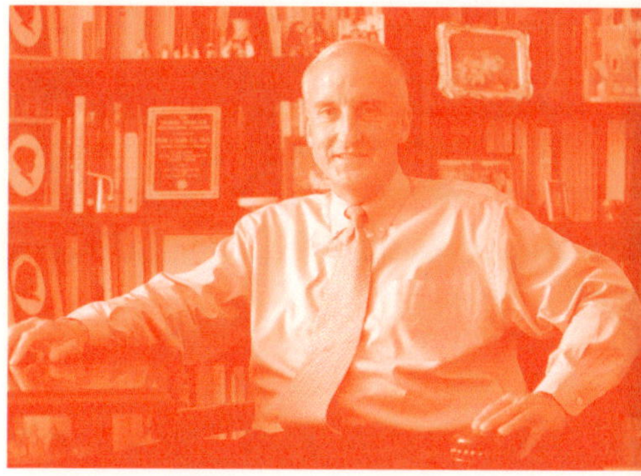

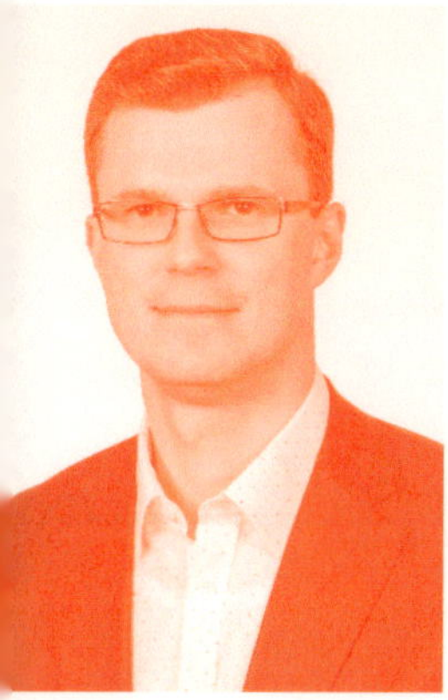

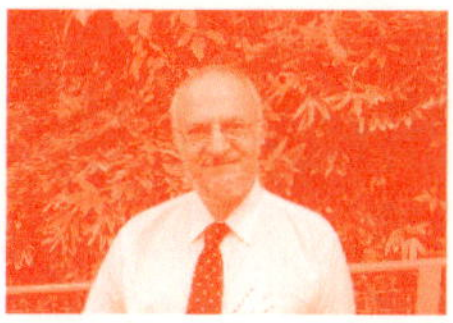

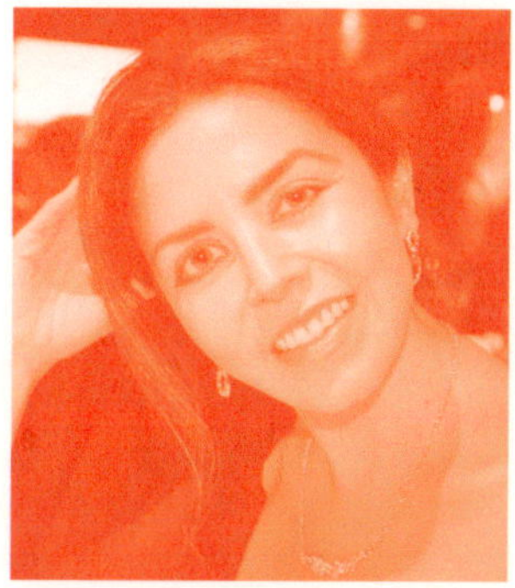

Supporting open minds since 2005

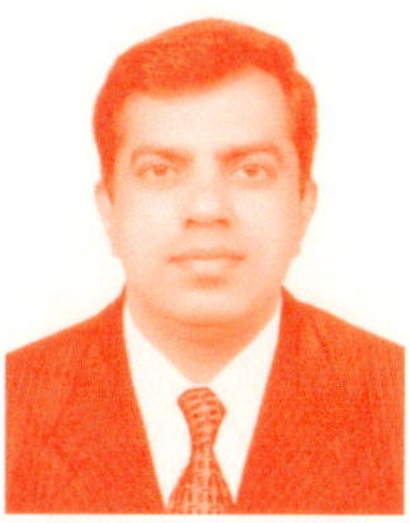

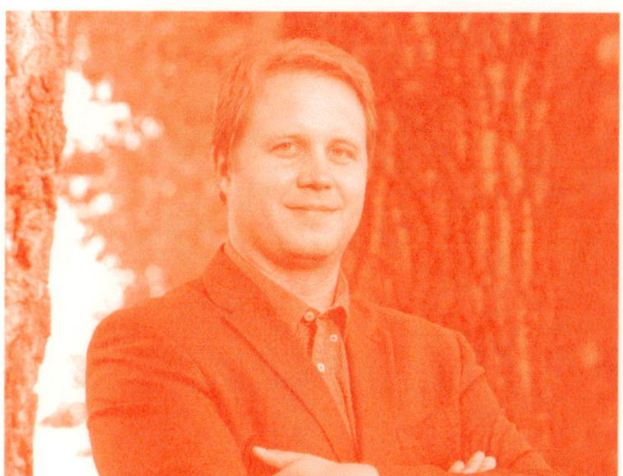

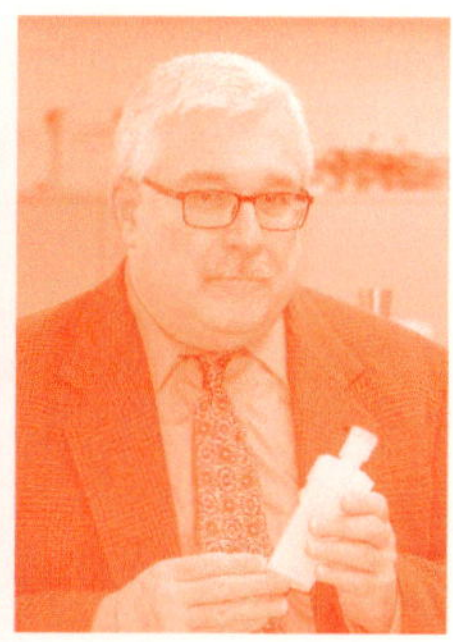

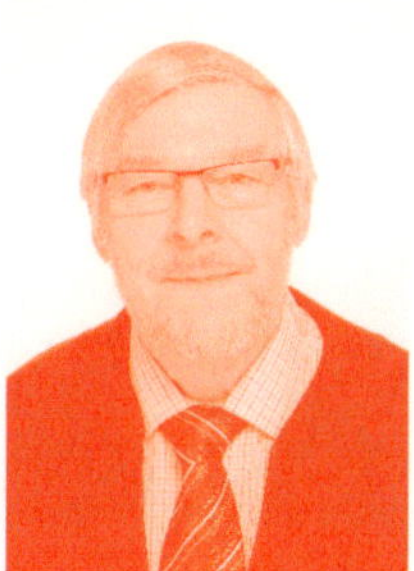

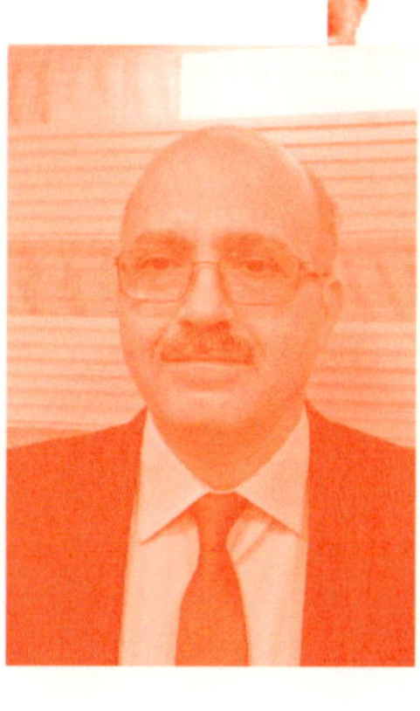

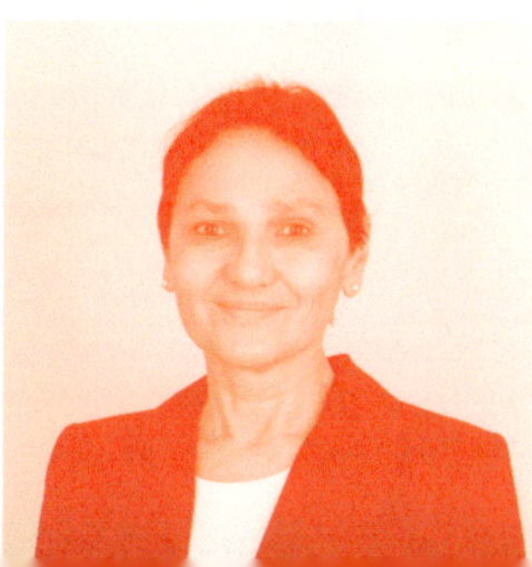

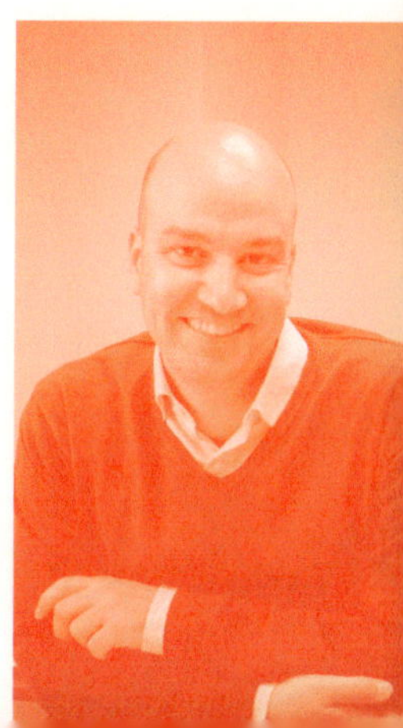

Amyloidosis - History and Perspectives
http://dx.doi.org/10.5772/intechopen.83041
Edited by Jonathan S. Harrison

Contributors
Nisha Arenja, Eva Strickler, Ernest Tsiaze, Gerrit Hellige, Dominik Zumstein, Dominik Waldmeier, Jonathan S. Scott Harrison, Irina Ioffe, Yossi Cohen, Shlomo Bulvik, Ivo Ilvan Kerppers, Andressa Panegalli Hosni, Andressa Leticia Miri, Ana Carolina Dorigoni Bini, Maria Elvira Ribeiro Cordeiro, Mariane Maria Silveira Vieira De Lima, Larissa Sakis Bernardi, Paulo Renato de Oliveira, Flávio Klinpovous Kerppers, Eliane Gonçalves De Jesus Fonseca, Patricia Pacheco Tyski Suckow, Felipe Figueiredo Moreira, Gilad A. Muth, Rohan Arora, Richa Juneja, Prasad Dange, Rahul Arora, Ivetta Danylesko

First published in London, United Kingdom, 2022 by IntechOpen
IntechOpen is the global imprint of INTECHOPEN LIMITED, registered in England and Wales, registration number: 11086078, 5 Princes Gate Court, London, SW7 2QJ, United Kingdom
Printed in Croatia

British Library Cataloguing-in-Publication Data
A catalogue record for this book is available from the British Library

Additional hard and PDF copies can be obtained from orders@intechopen.com

Amyloidosis - History and Perspectives
Edited by Jonathan S. Harrison
p. cm.
Print ISBN 978-1-83969-297-0
Online ISBN 978-1-83969-298-7
eBook (PDF) ISBN 978-1-83969-299-4

For EU product safety concerns:
IN TECH d.o.o., Prolaz Marije Krucifikse Kozulić 3, 51000 Rijeka, Croatia, info@intechopen.com or visit our website at intechopen.com.

Meet the editor

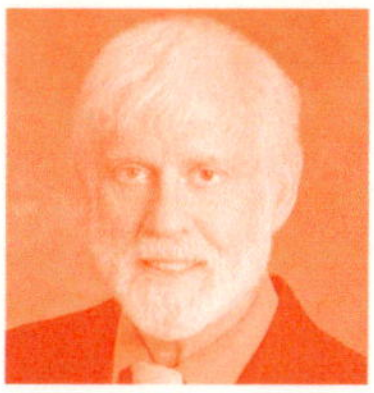

Jonathan S. Harrison obtained undergraduate and graduate degrees at the University of Chicago, prior to receiving his medical degree from the University of Illinois. Much of his career was spent in the medical education system of the State of New Jersey, which is now part of Rutgers University. He was subsequently the Nellie B. Smith Professor of Oncology and director of the division of Hematology and Oncology, University of Missouri. Currently, he is a member of the Hemato-Oncology Institute at the Sheba Medical Center.

Contents

Preface

Amyloidosis occurs in a variety of clinical settings and can manifest in a wide spectrum of clinical presentations. It may occur as an inherited disease or it may be acquired during the lifetime of the affected individual due to a variety of underlying disease states. As a consequence of heterogenous etiologies and of the protean clinical presentations, it is often overlooked until irreversible end-organ damage has occurred. This volume provides an overview of some of the major topics in the very broad field of amyloidosis to aid in the understanding of the nature of amyloidoses.

The first chapter provides a historical overview of the key developments in the understanding of amyloidosis with respect to biology and diagnosis as well milestones in the treatment of the major subtypes of the disease. Subsequent chapters focus on a variety of subtypes of amyloidosis and provide more detailed discussions of the pathogenesis of specific forms of amyloidosis as well as examine treatment options for these subtypes. The final chapter discusses major hypotheses regarding the role of amyloid in Alzheimer's disease, a disorder that is a major healthcare issue worldwide but for which the details of its pathobiology remain to be fully elucidated and for which treatment is entirely unsatisfactory.

There are medical journals devoted largely or entirely to amyloidosis and therefore one may ask what the role of yet another volume on the topic might be. New insights are being gleaned into the varied subtypes of amyloidosis yearly, and current updates are of value in stimulating thought and moving the basic and clinical investigation forward. More fundamentally, if even one patient ultimately benefits from the works contained herein, then this present volume may be judged a success.

This book is dedicated to George P. Studzinski, MD, Ph.D., Professor Emeritus, Rutgers University, a meticulous scientist, an accomplished educator, and an exemplary mentor.

Jonathan S. Harrison
Hemato-Oncology Institute,
Sheba Medical Center – Tel HaShomer Hospital,
Ramat Gan, Israel

Chapter 1

An Historical Overview of the Amyloidoses

Jonathan S. Harrison, Yossi Cohen, Irina Ioffe and Shlomo Bulvik

Abstract

The amyloidoses are a heterogenous group of clinical disorders that share the common finding of the abnormal deposition of insoluble proteins into various organs, with the result that these proteinaceous deposits disrupt cellular function and impair the integrity of the organs involved. Most typically, the abnormal protein deposition is the consequence of abnormal three dimensional folding of the culprit protein. The abnormal folding of the protein, in turn, may be due to a germ line mutation, may be due to an acquired mutation, or may be due to a polymorphism or characteristic of a normal protein that leads to abnormal folding, precipitation, and deposition of the protein, particularly when that protein is expressed at unusually high levels for a prolonged period of time. The clinical manifestations of an amyloid disorder are the consequences of the array of organs involved, the extent of amyloid deposition, and co-morbid conditions present in the individual patient. The array of organs involved, and the extent of organ involvement, in turn, depend in large part on the specific protein that is responsible for the amyloid deposition, and the process driving that protein's production. In this chapter, a chronological overview is intended to summarize the critical insights into the patho-biology of amyloid accumulation of various types. These insights have allowed an improved understanding over time of the of the major subgroups and disease entities of the amyloidoses, leading to some degree of improvement in diagnosis and treatment outcomes. Unfortunately, as of this writing, treatment outcomes still remain poor for a large fraction of patients, and there is need for improvement in all aspects of the evaluation and management of these diseases.

Keywords: amyloidosis, biological subtypes, medical history

1. Introduction

The amyloidoses are a heterogenous group of clinical disorders that share the common finding of the abnormal deposition of insoluble proteins into various organs, with the re sult that these proteinaceous deposits disrupt cellular function and impair the integrity of the organs involved. Most typically, the abnormal protein deposition is the consequence of abnormal three dimensional folding of the culprit protein. The abnormal folding of the protein, in turn, may be due to a germ line mutation - in which case the disease is a hereditary amyloidosis; the abnormal folding may be due to an acquired mutation, for example a mutation resulting in a B cell lymphoproliferative disorder as is seen in AL amyoidosis, also termed primary amyloidosis - in which an excess of an abnormal immunoglobulin light chain misfolds and results in amyloid deposition; or may be due to a polymorphism in the culprit protein that leads to abnormal folding, then precipitation, and then deposition of the protein, particularly when that protein is expressed at unusually high levels for a prolonged time period, as in the subtype of amyloid diseases termed AA amyloidosis, or as in renal dialysis associated amyloidosis. The clinical manifestations of an amyloid disorder are the consequences of the array of organs involved, the extent of amyloid deposition, and co-morbid conditions present in the individual patient. The array of organs involved, and the extent of organ involvement, in turn, depend in large part on the specific protein that is responsible for the amyloid deposition, and the process driving that protein's production.

In this chapter, a chronological overview is intended to summarize the critical insights, over time, into the patho-biology of amyloid accumulation of various subtypes. These insights have allowed an improved understanding over time of the of the major subgroups and disease entities of the amyloidoses, leading to some degree of improvement in diagnosis and treatment outcomes. Unfortunately, as of this writing, treatment outcomes still remain poor for a large fraction of patients, and there is need for improvement in all aspects of the evaluation and management of these diseases.

2. Early observations

Robert Kyle, of the Mayo Clinic, a leading investigator in the field of amyloidosis over much of the past century, meticulously detailed early observations regarding cases suggestive of amyloid diseases documented in the medical literature, in a historical review that he published shortly after the turn of this century [1]. Kyle references reports by Theophili Bonetti, in Bonetti's work *Sepulchretum sive Anatomia Practica*, which is included in E. R. Long's book A History of Pathology [2]. Bonetti's reports includes descriptions of two autopsies with findings suggestive of amyloidosis. The earliest of these reports is that of Nicklaus Fontanus, from the year 1639, whose report was of an autopsy of a young man who had evidence of epistaxis, jaundice, and ascities, with gross pathology showing abnormalities of the liver and spleen. Kyle also cites the book by Schwartz [3] to note an autopsy report from the year 1818, by an investigator named Merat, who described "lardaceous" changes in the liver - that is, changes in the appearance of the liver that appeared to show infiltration of the liver by a substance resembling lard - porcine fat. Subsequently, George Budd, in 1852, described several patients with liver infiltration by an abnormal substance, and in his chemical analysis, using the techniques available at the time, he reported these contained a significant amount of albumin - that is, protein, measured at sixteen percent of the infiltrate, with only approximately six percent fat, despite its appearance. Two of the subjects in his series showed similar infiltration of the kidneys, a pattern consistent with current presentations of amyloidosis [4]. In 1814, Colin and Gaultier de Chaubry observed the blue color change seen when starch is stained using iodine together with sulfuric acid. The pathologist Rudolph Virchow applied the term "amyloid" in the year 1854 to characterize the brain structures corpora amylacea due to the color changes seen with the application of iodine, expressing the belief that there was a starch like substance present [5]. In 1842, Carl Rokitansky reported hepatomegaly with hepatic infiltration by a gelatinous material, in a series of autopsies of patients with tuberculosis or syphilis. This may have been the first report of AA amyloidosis in the setting of chronic inflammation and infection. Similarly, in the year 1867, H. Weber reported amyloidosis in a patient with myeloma, with amyloid having been identified in the heart, kidneys, and spleen, consistent with what is now termed AL amyloidosis [6].

In the late nineteenth century, dyes were being widely explored for use in a variety of biochemical investigations, including for use as histopathologic stains. The aniline dye Congo Red was developed in 1883, when Paul Böttinger, at the Bayer Company in Germany, synthesized the compound as a potential pH indicator [7]. In 1923, Bennhold reported administration of Congo Red by intravenous injection into humans [8]. He injected solutions of Congo Red into twenty-one healthy subjects, and into twenty-one patients with a variety of illnesses, including patients with amyloidosis. He noted that in patients with amyloidosis, Congo Red cleared from the blood significant faster than in healthy individuals or patients with other disease states. In that report, one patient with a diagnosis of amyloidosis died within a day of the injection of Congo Red; at autopsy, the liver and spleen appeared to have been stained red by the injected dye Congo Red. In addition, light microscopy of histopathologic slides demonstrated red staining. The observation that a so-called "apple-green birefringence" could be observed in tissue involved by amyloid deposition under polarized light microscopy was made in the mid-twentieth century, variously attributed to Missmahl, a student of Bennhold, and to Divry and Florkin [9]. Over the course of the twentieth century, the technique of Congo Red staining has been refined, and the chemical basis of the staining has been generally well characterized. In an excellent review, Yakupova and colleagues detail both the empiric data, as well as biochemical models, regarding Congo Red staining of amyloid, in the context of the knowledge of amyloid structure [10]. They detail the pitfalls involved in the use of Congo Red staining as a histopathologic test for amyloidosis, and summarize the literature, including a discussion of false positives and false negatives with regard to the accurate diagnosis of amyloidosis.

As X-ray diffraction became available as a technique to study submicroscopic structure, this technology was applied to the study of amyloid. Eanes and Glenner reported X-ray diffraction studies on amyloid filaments in the year 1968 [11], from which it appeared that amyloid is composed of polypeptide chains in a "cross β conformation". Less than a decade prior to that, Cohen and Calkins applied electron microscopy imaging to recognize that all subtypes of amyloid exhibit a non-branching fibrillary structure [12]. Bonar and colleagues refined the characterization of amyloid fibrils using X-ray diffraction to show that for amyloid fibrils, the cross β proteins - polypeptide chains that form β pleated sheets - the individual strands of each β sheet run perpendicular to the fibril axis, with 4.1 Å spacing [13]. Thus, by the 1960s, the general structure of amyloid had been defined, although the underlying pathophysiology of the various subtypes remained to be more completely elucidated.

In recent decades, the application of high performance liquid chromatography (HPLC) and mass spectroscopy (MS) to the analysis of amyloid specimens has greatly enhanced the ability to diagnosis patients as having specific subtypes of amyloidosis, and thus has allowed marked improvements in disease-directed treatments. Mass spectroscopy is an analytical technique that is used to measure the mass-to-charge ratio of ions. The results are typically presented as a mass spectrum, a plot of intensity as a function of the mass-to-charge ratio. Comparison of the results of analysis of a specimen to know materials assists in identification of the composition of the specimen. The scientific basis for the technology of mass spectroscopy began with the work of Eugene Goldstein and Wilhelm Wein in Germany at the end of the 19th century. It was developed into a practical tool by J.J. Thompson in England, and refined by Arthur Jeffrey Dempster and F.W. Aston in the early 20th century. Similarly, HPLC a technique in analytical chemistry used to separate, identify, and quantify each component in a sample that is presumed to be a mixture. The device pumps a highly pressurized liquid solvent containing the sample mixture through a column filled with a solid adsorbent material, and the components are thereby separated and may be identified by comparisons to know controls. Although conventional liquid chromatography is a technique that was developed much earlier, modern high pressure liquid chromatography matured in the 1960s and 1970s. Thus, the application of this technology to characterize amyloid deposits only began in the 1970s, as discussed later, regarding the work of Mark Pepys and colleagues in characterizing the amyloid P protein.

3. Insights into patho-biological subtypes and diagnosis

3.1 AA amyloidosis

As noted above, autopsy studies in the nineteenth century, as exemplified by the report by Rokitansky in 1842, mentioned above, established a relationship between chronic inflammatory diseases - such as tuberculosis and syphillis, and the development, in some of these cases, of amyloidosis. Earl P. Benditt, a pioneer in the field of amyloidosis, together with his colleague Nils Eriksen at the University of Washington, isolated, by gel electrophoresis, a protein that he initially named "amyloid of unknown origin" in the year 1961 [14], obtained from specimens of patients with "secondary" amyloidosis - that is, in patients with underlying chronic inflammatory diseases. A decade later, in 1971, Benditt and colleagues refined their identification of the amino acid structure of secondary amyloid, showing a specific sequence of amino acids at the N-terminus [15]. The following year, in 1972, Levin and colleagues reported the complete seventy-six amino acid protein sequence of an amyloid protein from a subject with secondary amyloidosis [16]. A number of other laboratories identified similar peptide sequences from specimens of secondary amyloidisis, differing slightly in length, but all sharing the same N-terminal sequence, and with lengths on the order of approximately seventy-six amino acids.

These then became known as AA amyloid, or amyloid A protein. In 1975, Linke and colleagues, using antibodies raised against amyloid A proteins, identified a serum substance that bound these antibodies. Ultimately, this 104 amino acid peptide was identified as the serum precursor to tissue amyloid A, and was named serum amyloid A, or, SAA. There is now a large body of literature detailing the biology of SAA; the SAA proteins are acute phase reactants, which are important both in lipid transport and in inflammation, and participate in the interactions between lipids and the inflammatory process. These molecules are also termed apolipoproteins, in view of the function that they fulfill in transporting lipids throughout the body. The genes for human serum amyloid A1 (SAA1) and human serum amyloid A2 protein (SAA2) map to the region of chromosome 11 p15.1, and are rapidly synthesized by hepatocytes and secreted into the blood in response to a variety of inflammatory stimuli. In experimental conditions, exposure to lipopolysaccharide from *streptococcus pneumonia* provokes a dramatic rise in SAA levels and is associated with chemotaxis of leukocytes as well as a cascade of other inflammatory responses. SAA3 appears to be a pseudo-gene, with no significant protein expression, and SAA4 is expressed constitutively in the liver. AA amyloid fibrils include deposition of SAA1 and. SAA2, and this typically occurs when a significant inflammatory process persists over a long period of time. An excellent recent review of the literature on the structure and biology of serum amyloid A was published by George Sach in the journal Molecular Medicine [17].

In parallel with studies that defined the identity and structure of the amyloid A proteins, during the 1960s a number of investigators identified a separate protein extracted from amyloid deposits, by exploiting antigenic properties, using antibodies to isolate and characterize this protein. Prominent among these investigators were Cathcart and Cohen, and their colleagues at Harvard Medical School [18]. In a series of experiments reported over several years, this protein was defined, and named amyloid P protein [19], also called in the literature amyloid P component. In the early 1970s, Mark Pepys in London developed a rabbit antibody to C reactive protein (CRP) that also precipitated second protein from serum; this proved to be serum amyloid P (SAP). Over the next two decades, it was discerned that both CRP and SAP are members of the same class, pentameric molecules that have been named pentraxins [20]. Pepys and colleagues reported the three dimensional structure of human SAP using X-ray crystallography in 1994, ultimately finding that this forms a flattened β "jelly roll" structure [21]. The gene for SAP in humans resides on chromosome 1 at locus 1q23.2. Human SAP avidly binds to chromatin, displacing H1 histones; this has suggested that SAP may play a role in modulating DNA biology [22]; however much remains to be determined in this regard. An evolving literature indicates that the so-called "short pentraxins", which include CRP and SAP, are participants in the innate immune response. There is data that both CRP and SAP interact with pathogens to activate leukocytes, as well as to regulate complement; this has been carefully reviewed in a paper by Cox, Pilling, and Gomer of the University of Texas [23]. On average, approximately fourteen percent of the mass of amyloid deposits are amyloid P protein, across amyloid subtypes. In 1979, Pepys and colleagues demonstrated that, in vitro, amyloid P protein binds to both primary amyloid (immunoglobulin light chain amyloid), or AL amyloid, as noted above, as well as binding to secondary amyloid, such as AA amyloid. The amyloid P component is thought to stabilize other fibrillary molecules within the amyloid, such as the amyloid A protein, and inhibit fibril breakdown. Analysis of amyloid deposits by high performance liquid chromatography and mass spectroscopy has become an important tool in confirming the specific subtype of amyloidosis in a patient; a biopsy specimen processed by laser micro dissection can generally be sent to a reference laboratory for such analysis [24]. Such analysis permits determination and confirmation of the specific subtype of amyoidosis; e.g., that a particular specimen contains AA amyloid, AL amyloid, ATTR amyloid, or a less common subtype among the amyloidoses. This mass spectroscopy and high performance chromatography analysis has demonstrated the presence of other moieties present in amyloid deposits, prominently including glycos-aminoglycans, in addition to the ubiquitous amyloid P protein.

In the late 1980s, Pepys and colleagues developed the diagnostic technique of radioactive iodine labeled SAP scintigraphy for diagnosis and evaluation of patients with various forms of amyloidosis [25]. This diagnostic modality remains an important tool to this day in the assessment of patients with suspected to documented amyloidosis, including for the purpose of monitoring response to therapy.

In 2007, researchers in the United Kingdom published the findings of a longitudinal study of 374 patients with AA amyloidosis followed at the Royal Free hospital [26]. They reported that median survival from diagnosis was 133 months, and kidney dysfunction was the predominant clinical manifestation. They further reported that mortality and renal impairment correlated positively with SAA serum concentrations. In this series, underlying chronic inflammatory disorders included chronic inflammatory arthritis most commonly - predominantly Rheumatoid arthritis, chronic infections including bronchiectasis, infections in the setting of chronic injection drug abuse, and infectious complications of paraplegia. Less common underlying inflammatory processes included osteomyelitis, tuberculosis, and periodic fever syndromes such as familial Mediterranean fever; Crohn's disease, and Castleman's disease. Successful management of the underlying inflammatory disorder was associated with improved outcome and lower levels of SAA in the blood.

3.2 AL amyloidosis

Robert Kyle of the Mayo Clinic has published several historical reviews of the disease multiple myeloma. In a manuscript detailing medical observations and insights regarding myeloma, Kyle and Rajkumar [27] cite a case reported in the year 1844, of a 39 year old woman who experienced fatigue and bone pain associated with multiple fractures [28]. The patient died approximately four years after her initial presentation, and autopsy findings included marrow replacement by aberrant cells. A landmark case was that of the patient Thomas McBean, who also developed fatigue and bone pain. Urine specimens from Mr. McBean were brought to Henry Bence Jones, a chemical pathologist, after the patient's attending physician noted a high specific gravity to the urine, as well as opacity of the urine when boiled. Bence Jones reported the findings of proteinuria [29, 30], although he considered that the protein was an oxidized albumin. Waldeyer was the first to use the term plasma cell to describe a specific cell type [31]; however, it was Wright who felt that the malignant cells of myeloma were plasma cells [32]. H. Weber, in 1867, reported an autopsy with findings of non-traumatic fractures of the sternum, with the marrow replaced by an infiltrate of small uncleared cells. The heart was hypertrophied, and amyloid was identified in both the kidneys and the spleen - a presentation consistent with myeloma complicated by amyloidosis [33]. Kyle writes that this was the first report of amyloidosis associated with multiple myeloma. During the first half of the twentieth century, technology evolved to permit the identification of different classes of Bence Jones proteins, and in 1962, Edelman and Gally showed that serum monoclonal light chains from a patient with IgG myeloma shared the same amino acid sequence as the patient's Bence Jones protein, establishing that Bence Jones protein is derived from clonal paraprotein [34].

Magnus-Levy, who began his career in Germany, but relocated to the United States early during the Second World War, documented his conjecture that Bence Jones protein excreted in the urine of myeloma patients might be “the mother substance” of amyloidosis; this was published in the year 1931 [35]. In 1946, Herbut and Erf showed that amyloid could be identified within plasma cells, and concluded corrrectly that plasma cells were the source of amyloid in the setting of myeloma [36]. Thus, by the mid-twentieth century, it was evident that one form of amyloidosis was the consequence of a clonal plasma cell disorder. Glenner and colleagues demonstrated *in vitro* that monoclonal immunoglobulin light chains from myeloma patients could form amyloid fibrils under experimental conditions, which precipitated after pepsin exposure; the precipitates stained with Congo Red, and demonstrated green birefringence by polarizing microscopy [37]. In the past several decades, it has been shown that specific clonal light chain sequences result in a significant predisposition to misfold, and therefore deposit as amyloid; among these, the light chain variable region sequences Vλ1, Vλ2, Vλ3, Vλ6, and Vκ1 are particularly over-represented as amyloid protein, as compared to other immunoglobulin variable region sequences [38].

The treatment of primary, or, AL amyloidosis remains unsatisfactory. This is, in part, due to a frequent delay in diagnosis, which may result either from the lack of specificity in early symptoms, or due to presentation when there is already significant end-organ damage that precludes aggressive therapy [39]. Treatment of all subtypes of amyloidosis are directed, at least in part, to suppressing production of the misfolding protein. In AL amyloidosis, this means suppressing production of clonal light chains secreted by the clonal plasma cells. In 1958, Blokhin and colleagues reported benefit from treatment using melphalan in a small cohort of patients [40]. Similarly, in 1962, Maas reported a study in myeloma patients treated using prednisone, versus placebo, and documented the at least transient objective anti-neoplastic activity of corticosteroid therapy in treating myeloma [41]. In 1969, Alexanian and colleagues published a seminal prospective, randomized clinical trial that established the combination of melphalan and prednisone as the standard of care as systemic anti-neoplastic therapy for multiple myeloma [42]. That standard prevailed for several decades, until the turn of this century, when novel agents, including the imids and subsequently the proteosome inhibitors, were developed. Consequently, in view of the ability of theses drugs to suppress the malignant clone of plasma cells in overt myeloma, the same drugs were employed to suppress the clonal plasma cell population producing amyloid in AL amyloidosis. Toward the end of the twentieth century, colchicine was used as therapy for AL amyloidosis. However, a prospective, randomized clinical trial comparing colchicine to melphalan plus prednisone, or all three drugs together, in patients with AL amyloidosis, showed a survival advantage from melphalan and prednisone [43]. This was therefore conventional therapy for AL amyloidosis for several decades, until the advent of the newer agents used to treat multiple myeloma - the imids and proteosome inhibitors, and the demonstration that a favorable outcome - as compared to historical controls - could be obtained in carefully selected patients treated using high dose melphalan with autologous hematopoietic rescue. To date, there have been no large, prospective randomized clinical trials in AL amyloidosis of the newer agents, nor of autologous transplants in AL amyloidosis. However, based on numerous Phase II trials, a general consensus has evolved, with patients deemed fit taken to autologous transplant, often after induction therapy. One example of such a consensus approach is an algorithm for treatment published by the Swiss Amyloidosis Network [44]. This group currently recommends induction therapy using the combination of cyclophosphamide, bortezomib, and dexamethasone ("CyBorD") followed by high dose melphalan with autologous hematopoietic rescue, for transplant-eligible patients. For transplant ineligible patients, this group recommends the monoclonal antibody daratumumab, directed against the plasma cell surface protein CD 38, either alone or with combination with other agents. Current investigational therapeutic approaches include novel experimental treatments, such as a monoclonal antibody that can bind and potentially extract amyloid P protein from organ deposits [45].

3.3 ATTR amyloidosis

In 1952, a neurologist, Andrade, reported detailed observations regarding a cluster of patients with neurological deficits in the Oporto region of Portugal, with some of those observations dating back to 1939 [46]. The afflicted patients shared clinical features of peripheral motor weakness and peripheral sensory deficits, as well as, in many cases, gastrointestinal and sexual dysfunction. Histopathologic examination revealed amyloid deposition, and a familial, autosomal dominant pattern of inheritance was noted. Similar observations were made of familial amyloidosis with primarily neurological manifestations - most prominently peripheral neuropathy and autonomic neuropathy - in Japan, and in Scandinavia in the latter part of the twentieth century. Eventually, hereditary amyloidosis was identified in many populations, with clinical syndromes that presented primarily as neurological dysfunction, or with clinical syndromes that presented primarily with cardiac disease. Abnormal electrophoretic mobility transthyretin was noted in many of these cases. With the advent of the technologies of molecular biology of the gene, the vast majority of hereditary amyloidosis cases were found to be due to a variety of mutations in the protein transthyretin became recognized. Hereditary transthyretin amyloidosis, also termed ATTRv amyloidosis ("ATTR variant") is generally an autosomal dominantly inherited disorder, due to a variety of mutations in the

TTR gene that encodes for transthyretin. The TTR gene product is a homodimeric plasma protein produced primarily in the liver, with additional production and secretion by the choroid plexus and by retinal epithelia. The TTR protein serves both as a thyroid hormone binding protein, as well as a retinol binding protein, and was originally called “pre-albumin” due to its migratory pattern on protein gel electrophoresis, running ahead of the albumin peak [47]. Beginning in the late 1980s into the early 1990s, DNA sequencing of the TTR gene by many investigators uncovered numerous mutations in TTR associated with amyloidosis, manifesting as predominantly either neurological disease, or as cardiac disease- typically with arrhythmia, with or without heart failure syndrome [48]. As of this writing, more than 125 different TTR mutations have been identified in the TTR gene locus, that are associated with ATTR amyloidosis. The most common TTR variants in the United States include (1) the Val30Met mutation, which is the most commonly identified mutation worldwide. The syndrome Familial amyloid polyneuropathy (termed FAP) is most commonly caused by Val30Met. Other relatively common driver mutations include (2) the Thr60Ala mutation, (3) the Leu58His mutation, (4) the Ser77Tyr mutation, and (5) the Val122Ile mutation. This last mutation is predominantly seen in the African-American population, and typically presents as cardiomyopathy. The syndrome Familial Amyloid Cardiomyopathy (FAC) is commonly caused by Val122lle.

During the same time period, it was recognized, primarily from autopsy studies, that there were individuals who were found to have evidence of systemic amyloid deposition at an advanced age, primarily in the heart, but in some cases affecting the peripheral nerves, and this has been termed Systemic Senile Amyloidosis (SSA). Often there is no clinical heart disease in these individuals, but some of these individuals will indeed develop cardiac disease, ranging from arrhythmia to heart failure syndrome. There is also increasing evidence that ATTRwt disease is a cause of carpel tunnel syndrome in the elderly. Analysis of the amyloid from these patients showed transthyretin as the major component of the amyloid, together with serum amyloid A protein; there is also data to suggest that the molecule Clusterin may play a role in the formation of this form of amyloid [49]. Clusterin, also called apolipoprotein J, is a heterodimeric protein member of the heat shock protein family, and participates in apoptosis. Critically, gene sequencing of the TTR in these individuals is normal, as was first documented in a study by Westermark and colleagues in 1990 [50]. This subtype of ATTR amyloidosis is also termed ATTRwt, that is, wild-type ATTR Amyloidosis. In this disorder, there is misfolding of transthyretin, despite the normal gene sequence.

When ATTR amyloidosis is suspected due to clinical findings, a tissue diagnosis of amyloid deposition is a definitive procedure. The finding of amyloid deposition, however, should be followed by biochemical analysis of the amyloid, either by mass spectroscopy and high performance chromatography, or by sequencing of the TTR gene, or both. As noted above, ATTRwt is defined in part by a normal gene sequence of TTR. As discussed previously, as in all subtypes of systemic amyloidosis, nuclear medicine studies may be diagnostic [25, op cit]. Myocardial radiotracer uptake at bone scintigraphy using an agent such as technicium-99 pyrophosphate is both sensitive and specific for a diagnosis of cardiac amyloid due to ATTR amyloid, once monoclonal light chain amyloid has been excluded by immunological studies. In the management of ATTRv amyloidosis, liver transplant became a standard of care over the past 25 years, as this replaces the source of the variant, or, mutated TTR with a liver that produces normal TTR. Liver transplant has been documented to improve overall survival in ATTRv amylodosis [51]. In ATTRv amyloidosis, the mutations in the TTR gene appear to destabilize the normal tetrameric state of the transthyretin protein, resulting in dissociation into monomers prone to misfolding and aggregating. Consequently, it was hypothesized that agents that could stabilize the TTR tetramers might ameliorate the disease by reducing amyloid fibril formation and deposition. Tafamidis is an oral agent, currently approved in Europe for the treatment of early stage polyneuropathy ATTR amyloidosis, which appears to work by stabilizing the transthyretin tetramer. In prospective, randomized clinical trials, Tafamidis was shown to be safe, with evidence of that it retards neurological deterioration [52, 53]; however efficacy was questionable for patients with advanced disease. Subsequently, a prospective, randomized, placebo controlled trial of Tafamidis in ATTR cardiomyopathy, both variant and wild type, NCT01994889, showed a thirty percent reduction in mortality as compared to placebo [54]. This led to FDA approval in the United States of Tafamidis for the treatment of ATTR cardiomyopathy. In a randomized, placebo controlled clinical trial, the non-steroidal anti-inflammatory agent diflunisal was compared to placebo, diflunisal reduced progression of neuropathy significantly in patients with hereditary ATTR amyloidosis [55]. However, there were significant toxicities associated with use of diflunisal, including renal injury, in this study. Use of diflunisal is "off-label", but is certainly used at this time for management of some patients with ATTRv amyloidosis.

More recently, two parenteral agents have been introduced for the treatment of ATTR amyloidosis with polyneuropathy, both of which work by reducing messenger RNA for TTR, and thus reducing production of the amyloidogenic TTR protein. Inotersen, an anti-sense oligonucleotide that binds up TTR mRNA, is administered subcutaneously once weekly, and was approved on the basis of the results of a pivotal randomized clinical trial. In that study, the Neuro-TTR trial, patients randomized to Inotersen demonstrated sustained reductions in transthyretin protein production, and statistically significant improvement in quality of life [56]. Similarly, Patisiran is a small, interfering RNA molecule given intravenously once every three weeks. In the Apollo study, patients with hereditary ATTR polyneuropathy were randomized to receive Patisiran versus placebo. Results documented a clinical improvement in neuropathy at eighteen months for patients treated using Patisiran versus placebo [57]. Both Inotersen and Patisiran are currently approved for treatment of ATTR polyneuropathy. In sum, for the estimated 50,000 people living with hereditary ATTR amyloidosis, there are now a number of medical treatment options with less mortality risk than liver transplant.

4. Other hereditary amyloidosis

Since 1990, several other molecules with mutations that predispose to misfolding have been discovered as rare causes of amyloidosis. These include hereditary renal amyloidosis due to mutations in lysozyme [58] giving rise to ALys Amyloidosis; mutations in fibrinogen, giving rise to AFib amyloidosis [59] apolipoproteins AI, giving rise to AApoAI amyloidosis; mutations in Apolipoprotein AII, giving rise to AApoAII amyloidosis [60]; mutations in the protein gelsolin, giving rise to AGel amyloidosis [61].

In addition, leukocyte chemotactic factor-2 related amyloidosis is an unusual amyloid disorder associated primarily with chronic kidney disease. Originally characterized in 1998, human LECT2 is a protein that is predominantly synthesized by hepatocytes. As well as having neutrophil chemotactic properties, it also appears to participate in repair of tissue injury. Since the beginning of the 21st century, an increasing number of cases of patients with localized renal amyloidosis associated with chronic kidney disease have been found, on chemical analysis, to have amyloid comprised largely of LECT2. There is a marked over-representation of Hispanic patients with LECT2 amyloidosis, in particular patients with backgrounds from Mexico. Although the majority of these unusual cases have renal involvement only, investigators at the University of California reported a case with both renal and pulmonary involvement [62]. Genetic polymorphisms in the LECT2 gene have been identified that appear to predispose to the development of amyloidosis, and the over-representation of Hispanic patients suggests that there is a genetic component to this disease process. However, the precise etiology of the over-expression and deposition of LECT2 has not been fully established as of this writing.

5. Dialysis associated amyloidosis

Dialysis-related amyloidosis ("DRA") is a relatively common complication of chronic renal dialysis therapy, with the deposition of amyloid fibrils that are composed primarily of the molecule β2 microglobulin ("β2M"). β2M is typically hydrogen bonded to the MHC class I structure present on nucleated cell surfaces, but urea in the blood can break that bond, with β2M then circulating in the plasma. In 1975, carpel tunnel syndrome was recognized as a complication of long term hemodialysis [63]. Within a decade, this was found to be associated with histology findings of amyloid [64], and β2M was found to accumulate in patients maintained on dialysis. Soon thereafter, the amyloid deposits seen in this setting were documented to be composed in large part of β2M [65]. The amyloid in the setting of chronic renal dialysis therapy is deposited in osteoporosis-articular structures and in visceral organs, particularly at the wrists, the sternum, the knees, and the kidneys. Bone cysts also occur. Under normal physiological conditions, β2M is eliminated through glomerular filtration and subsequent reabsorption and catabolism by the proximal tubules. In general, the serum level of β2M is inversely related to the glomerular filtration rate; therefore, in end-stage renal disease patients, β2M levels may increase up to 60-fold. The β2M may then mis-fold, polymerize, and become deposited in the tissues; mis-folded intermediate forms of β2M have been reported [66], particularly truncated forms of β2M that lack the six N-terminal amino acids [67]. It is difficult to determine the true prevalence of DRA, because formal evaluation is often not undertaken. DRA is relatively common in patients maintained on long-term hemodialysis, typically for at least several years, but it has also been documented in patients undergoing continuous ambulatory Peritoneal dialysis. Aggressive dialysis, to reduce the chronic elevation of β2M is a costly, but effective, management approach.

Instances of localized deposition of amyloid – as distinct from systemic amyloidosis – were clearly recognized as a distinct clinical entity only in the twentieth century. Among the earliest reports of localized amyloid deposition is that by Gellerstedt in the year 1938 [68]. He described Congo Red positive amyloid deposits in the islets of langerhans within the pancreas, in a diabetic patient. Since that time, localized amyloidosis has been reported to occur, in rare cases, in nearly every organ in humans. However, the most commonly reported sites, by far, are the skin and the upper aero-digestive tract. Weidner and colleagues from Germany reviewed the literature regarding localized cutaneous amyloidosis, and identified small case series and case reports dating back to the year 1985 [69]. Similarly, the upper aero-digestive tract is a relatively frequent site for identification of localized amyloid deposits, in the absence of systemic disease. However, these cases are still fairly rare overall, in general, and information regarding localized amyloidosis of the upper aero-digestive tract is primarily derived from case reports and small series [70]. It is possible that the medical literature may be skewed, and upper aero-digestive tract amyloid deposits may be over-represented, due to the fact that mass lesions in the upper aero-digestive tract give rise to symptoms even when the lesions are quite small, but there are a relatively large number of case reports of localized amyloid in the regions from the oropharynx to the pulmonary carina. In a retrospective review from Germany, the larynx was the most commonly involved site, although in that series localized disease was also seen in the tongue, trachea, and pharynx [71]. Similarly, there are many reports of localized amyloid in the lower gastrointestinal tract, likely due in part to incidental discovery during screening colonoscopy for colon cancer. An early autopsy series reported by Ravid and colleagues, published in the year 1967, detailed the findings from 391 necropsies performed at Tel HaShomer Hospital [68, op cit]. Most cases of localized amyloidosis are found to be AL amyloid, but AA amyloid may also be seen. It remains unclear why some patients with localized AL amyloid may not progress to systemic amyloid, nor why there is a tropism for the amyloid deposition to the specific sites in such cases. This is a fertile area for additional research.

6. Cerebral vascular amyloidosis

Cerebral amyloid angiopathy is a disorder in which there is accumulation of amyloid within the walls capillaries, as well as of small and medium sized arterial vessels within the nervous system. This results in weakening of the vessels over time, and the disorder typically presents in the elderly. Clinically, it may manifest as either micro-hemorrhages, which can result in cognitive impairment and possibly vascular dementia, or may manifest as intra-cerebral hemorrhage, which may be catastrophic. An early description of cerebral amyloid angiopathy was published by Ishiguro and colleagues in the year 1984. In this autopsy series, the authors identified seven cases in which patients presented with either intra-cerebral hemorrhage or with dementia. At autopsy, amyloid deposition was observed in the smaller arterial vessels, including at the sites of hemorrhage [72]. Later analysis of the amyloid showed this to be deposition of Amyloid Precursor Protein (APP), a membrane protein that is present in high concentrations at neuronal synapses. Proteolysis of APP results in amyloid Aβ polypeptides. These are a principle component of the amyloid found in cerebral vascular amyloidosis; amyloid Aβ polypeptide is also a component of the amyloid deposits in Alzheimer's Disease. However, in Alzheimer's Disease, the Aβ fragments typically extend to amino acids position 42, whereas in cerebral vascular amyloidosis, the Aβ fragments extend only to amino acid positions 39 or 40 [73]. Neurofibrillary tangles, a hallmark of Alzheimer's Disease, are not seen in cerebral vascular amyloidosis.

7. Amyloid in Alzheimer's disease

Amyloid deposition is an integral aspect of the histopathology of Alzheimer's Disease. However, the amyloid is only one aspect of the dramatic microscopic changes seen in the brain when affected by Alzheimer's disease. Alzheimer's disease is discussed in detail in other chapters of this volume, and therefore will not be reviewed here. A timeline of the many of the most significant observations and developments in the amyloidoses is provided in **Figure 1**.

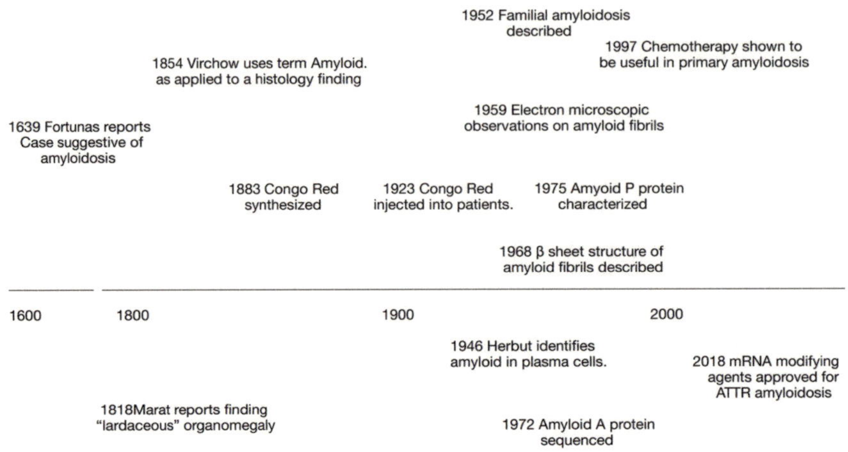

Figure 1.
A timeline of major developments in Amyloidosis.

Author details

Jonathan S. Harrison[1,2]*, Yossi Cohen[2], Irina Ioffe[2] and Shlomo Bulvik[2]

1 Rutgers University, Newark, New Jersey, USA

2 Laniado Hospital, Netanya, Israel

*Address all correspondence to: jsharrisonmd@gmail.com

References

[1] Kyle, R. Amyloidosis: a convoluted story. 2001 Brit J Haematology Vol 114, p 529-538

[2] Bonetti, T. Sepulchretum sive Anatomia Practica ex cadaveribus Moro denatis cited in: E. Long, editor, A History of Pathology (1928) Williams & Wilkins, Baltimore

[3] Schwartz P. (1970) Amyloidosis: Causes and Manifestations of Senile Deterioration Charles C. Thomas, Springfield, Illinois

[4] Budd G. (1852) On Diseases of the Liver. 2nd edition, J. Churchill, London, UK

[5] Virchow R (1971) Lecture XVII. Amyloid degeneration. Inflammation. In: Cellular Pathology as based upon Physiologic and Pathological Histology. Dover Publications, New York

[6] Weber, H (1867) Mollities ossium, doubtful whether carcinomatous or syphilitic. Transactions of the Pathological Society of London. Vol 18, p 206-210

[7] Steensma D (2001) “Congo” red: out of Africa? Arch Pathol Lab Vol 125, p 250-252

[8] Bennhold H (1922) Specific staining of amyloid by Congo Red.MuEnchener Medizinische Wachenschrift. Vol 69, p 1537-1538

[9] Divry P and Florkin M (1927) Sur Les proprietés optiques de l’amyloid. Competes Rendux des Sèances de la Societè de Biologie et de ses Filialis Vol 97, p 1808-1810

[10] Yakupova EL, Bobyleva LG, Vikhlyantsev IM, Bobylev AG. Congo Red and amyloid: history and relationship (2019) Bioscience Reports Vol 39, p 1-23

[11] Eanes ED, and Glenner GG. (1968) X-ray diffraction studies on amyloid filaments. J Histochem Cytochemistry Vol 16, p 673-677

[12] Cohen AS and Calkins E (1959) Electron microscopic observations on a fibrous component in amyloid of diverse origins. Nature Vol 183, p 1202-1203

[13] Bonar L, Cohen AS, Skinner MM (1969) characterization of the amyloid fibril as a cross beta protein. Proc Soc Exp Biol Med Vol 131, p 1373-1375

[14] Benditt EP, Eriksen N. (1961) Starch gel electrophoresis of some proteins extracted from amyloid. Arch Path. Vol 78, p 326-330

[15] Benditt EP, Eriksen N, Hermonson MA, Ericsson LH (1971) The major proteins of human and monkey amyloid substance: Common properties including unusual N-terminal amino acid sequences. FEBS Letters Vol 19, p 169-173

[16] Levin M, Franklin EC, Frangione B, Pras M. (1972) The amino acid sequence of a major non immunoglobulin component of some amyloid fibrils. J Clinical Inv Vol 51, p 2773-2775

[17] Sach, GH. Serum amyloid A - a review. (2018) Molecular Medicine Vol 24, p 46-73

[18] Cathcart ES, Comerford FR, Cohen AS. (1965) Immunologic studies on a protein extracted from human secondary amyloid. N England J Med Vol 273, p 143-146

[19] Cathcart ES, Skinner M, Cohen AS, et al. (1970) Antigenic determinants in amyloid deposits. Nature Vol 228, p 1090-1091

[20] Osmand AP, Friedenson B, Gewurz H, et al. (1977)

Characterization of C-reactive protein and the complement subcomponent C1t as homologous proteins displaying cyclic pentameric symmetry (pentraxins). PNAS Vol 74, p 739-743

[21] Ashton AW, Boehm MK, Gallimore JR, et al. (1997) Pentameric and Decameron structures in solution of serum amyloid P component by X-ray and neutron scattering and molecular modeling analysis. J Mol Biol Vol 272, p 408-422

[22] Butler PJG, Tennent GA, Pepys MB (1990) Pentraxin-chromatin interactions: serum amyloid P component specifically displaces H1-type histones and solubilizes native long chromatin. J Exp Med Vol 172, p 13-18

[23] Cox N, Pilling D, Gomer RH (2014) Serum amyloid P: a systemic regulator of the innate immune response. J Leuk Biol Vol 96, p 739-743

[24] Vrana JA, Gamez JD, Madden BJ, et al. (2009) Classification of amyloidosis by laser micro dissection and mass spectrometry based proteomics analysis in clinical biopsy specimens. Blood Vol 114, p 4957-4959

[25] Hawkins PN, Lavender JP, Pepys MB (1990) Evaluation of systemic amyloidosis by scintigraphy with 131-I labeled serum amyloid P component. N England J Med Vol 323, p 508-513

[26] Lachmann HJ, Goodman HJB, Gilbertson JA, et al (2007) Natural history and outcome in systemic AA amyloidosis. N England J Med Vol 356, p 2361-2371

[27] Kyle RA and Rajkumar SV (2008) Multiple myeloma. Blood Vol 111, p 2962-2972

[28] Solly S (1844) Remarks on the pathology of mollities osseum with cases. Med Chir Trans London Vol 27, p 435-461

[29] Bence Jones H (1847) Chemical pathology. Lancet Vol 2, p 88-92

[30] Bence Jones H (1848) On the new substance in the urine of a patient with mollities osseum. Philos Trans R Soc London Vol 148, p 55-62

[31] Waldeyer W (1875) Ueber bindegewebszellen. Arch Microbiol Anat Vol 11, p 176-194

[32] Wright JH (1900) A case of multiple myeloma. Trans Assoc Am Phys Vol 15, p 137-147

[33] Weber H (1867) Mollities osseum, doubtful whether carcinomatous or syphilitic. Transact Patholog Society London Vol 18, p 206-210

[34] Edelman GM and Gally JA (1962) The nature of Bence Jones proteins: chemical similarities to polypeptide chains of myeloma globulins and normal gamma-globulins. J Exp Med Vol 116, p 207-227

[35] Magnus-Levy A. (1931) Bence-Jones-Eiweiss und amyloid. Zeitschrift für Klinische Medizinsche Vol 116, p 510-531

[36] Herbut PA, Erf LA (1946) Lipoblastic and megakarycytoid multiple myeloma. American J Clin Pathol Vol 16, p 13-21

[37] Glenner GG, Erin D, Eanes ED, et al (1971) Creation of 'amyloid' fibrils from Bence Jones protein *in vitro*. Science Vol 174, p 712-714

[38] Abraham RS, Geyer SM, Price-Troska TL, et al (2003) Immunoglobulin light chain variable (V) region genes influence clinical presentation and outcome in light-chain associated amyloidosis (AL) Blood Vol 101, p 3801-3808

[39] Merlini G, Dispenzieri A, Sanchorawala V, et al (2018) Systemic immunoglobulin light chain amyloidosis. Nat Rev Dis Primers Vol 4, p 38-46

[40] Blokhin N, Larionov L, Perevodchikova N, et al (1958) Clinical experiences with sarcolysin in neoplasticism diseases. Ann NY Acad Sci Vol 68, p 1128-1132

[41] Maas RE (1962) A comparison of the effect of prednisone and a placebo in the treatment of multiple myeloma. Cancer Chemother Rep Vol 16, p 257-259

[42] Alexanian R, Haut A, Khan AU, et al (1969) Treatment for multiple myeloma: combination chemotherapy with different melphalan dose regimens. JAMA Vol 208, p 1680-1685

[43] Kyle RA, Gertz MA, Greipp PR, et al (1997) A trial of three regimens for primary amyloidosis: colchicine alone, melphalan and prednisone, and melphalan, prednisone and colchicine. N England J Med Vol 336, p 1202-1207

[44] Schwatzer R, Flammer AJ, Gerull S, et al (2020) Expert recommendations from the Swiss Amyloidosis Network. Swiss Med Weekly Vol 150, w20364

[45] Van Doren L. and Lentzsch S. (2020) Nonchemotherapy Treatment of Immunoglobulin Light Chain Amyloidosis. Vol 143, p 373-380

[46] Andrade C (1952) A peculiar form of Peripheral neuropathy: familiar atypical general amyloidosis with special involvement of the peripheral nerves. Brain Vol 75, p 408-427

[47] Koike H, and Katsuno M. (2019) Ultrastructure in Transthyretin Amyloidosis: From Pathophysiology to Therapeutic Insights. Biomedicines Vol 7, p 11-27

[48] Nordlie M, Sletten K, Husby G, et al. (1988) A new prealbumin variant in familial amyloid cardiomyopathy of Danish origin. Scand J Immunol Vol 27, p 119-22

[49] Celia M. Torres-Arancivia CM, Chang D, Hackett WD, et al (2020) Glycosylation of Serum Clusterin in Wild-Type Transthyretin-Associated (ATTRwt) Amyloidosis: A Study of Disease-Associated Compositional Features Using Mass Spectrometry Analyses. Biochemistry Vol 59, p 4367-4378

[50] Westermark P, Sletten K, Johansson B (1990) Fibril in senile systemic amyloidosis is derived from normal transthyretin. Proc Natl Acad Sci USA. Vol 87, p 2843-2845

[51] Yamashita T, Ando Y, Okamoto S, et al. (2012) Long-term survival after liver transplantation in patients with familial amyloid polyneuropathy. Neurology Vol 78, p 637-643

[52] Coelho T, Maia LF, da Silva A, et al (2013) Long-term effects of tafamidid for the treatment of transthyretin familial amyloidosis polyneuropathy. J Neurology Vol 260, p 2803-2814

[53] Coelho T, Maia LF, da Silva A, et al (2012) Tafamidis for transthyretin familial amyloid polyneuropathy. Neurology Vol 79, p 785-792

[54] Li B, Alvin J, Stewart M (2020) Extrapolation of Survival Benefits in Patients with Transthyretin Amyloid Cardiomyopathy Receiving Tafamidis: Analysis of the Tafamidis in Transthyretin Cardiomyopathy Clinical Trial. Cardiol Ther Vol 9, p 535-540

[55] Berk JL, Suhr OB, Obici L, et al (2013) Repurposing diflunisal for familial amyloid polyneuropathy: A randomized clinical trial. JAMA Vol 310, p 2658-2667

[56] Benson MD, Waddington-Cruz M, Berk JL, et al (2018) Inotersen treatment for patients with hereditary transthyretin amyloidosis. N England J Med Vol 379, p 22-31

[57] Adams D, Gonzalez-Duarte A, O'Riordan WO, et al (2018) Evaluation of quality of life and disability in patients with hereditary transthyretin-mediated (hATTR) amyloidosis with polyneuropathy following treatment with Patisiran, an investigational RNAi therapeutic: Results from a phase 3 Apollo study. 70th Amer Acad Neurol annual meeting

[58] Li Z, Xu H, Lia D, et al. (2019) Hereditary renal amyloidosis with a variant lysozyme p.Trp82Arg in a Chinese family: case report and review of the literature. BMC Nephrology Vol 20, p 310-326

[59] Yazaki M, Yoshinaga T, Sekijima Y, et al (2018) Hereditary fibrinogen Aα chain amyloidosis in Asia: clinical and molecular characteristics. Int J Molecule Sciences Vol 19, p 320-330

[60] Valliex S, Verona G, Journey-Chiche N, et al. (2016) D25V apolipoprotein C-III variant causes dominant hereditary systemic amyloidosis and confers cardiovascular protective lipoprotein profile. Nature Commun Vol 7, p 10353-10355

[61] Solomon JP, Page LJ, Balch WE, Kelly JW (2012) Gelsolin Amyloidosis: Genetics, Biochemistry, Pathology and Possible Strategies for Therapeutic Intervention. Crit Rev Biochemical Molecule Biol Vol 47, p 282-296

[62] Khalighi M, Yue A, Hwang M-T, Wallace W. Leukocyte chemotactic factor 2 (LECT2) amyloidosis presenting as pulmonary-renal syndrome: a case report and review of the literature Clin Kidney J 2013 Vol 6, p 618-621

[63] Warren DJ, Otieno LS. (1975) Carpal tunnel syndrome in patients on intermittent haemodialysis. Postgrad Med J. Vol 51, p 450-452

[64] Fenves AZ, Emmett M, White MG, Greenway G. (1986) Carpal tunnel syndrome with cystic bone lesions secondary to amyloidosis in chronic hemodialysis patients. Am J Kidney Dis. Vol 7, p 130-134.

[65] Gejyo F, Yamada T, Odani S, et al. (1985) A new form of amyloid protein associated with chronic haemodialysis was identified as beta 2 microglobulin. Biochem Biophys Res Commun. Vol 129, p 701-706

[66] Heegaard NH, Sen JW, Kaarsholm NC, Nissen MH. (2001) Conformational intermediate of the amyloidogenic protein beta 2-microglobulin at neutral pH. J Biol Chem. Vol 276, p 32657-32662

[67] Eichner T, Kalverda AP, Thompson GS, Homans SW, Radford SE. (2011) Conformational conversion during amyloid formation at atomic resolution. Mol Cell. Vol 41, p 161-172.

[68] Ravid M, Gafni J, Sohar E, Missmahl HP. Incidence and origin of non-systemic microdeposits of amyloid. J Clin Pathol (1967) Vol 20, p 15-20

[69] Weidner T, Illing T, Elsner P. Primary localized cutaneous amyloidosis: A systematic treatment review. Am J Clin Dermatol 2017, Oct Vol 18, pp 629-642

[70] Pribitkin E, Friedman O, O'Hara B, et al. Amyloidosis of the upper aerodigestive tract. 2003 December Vol 113, p 2095-2101

[71] Send T, Spiegel J, Schade G, et al. Amyloidosis of the upper aerodigestive tract: Management of a rare disease and

review of the literature. 2019 Dysphagia Vol 34 pp 179-191

[72] Ishii N, Nishihara Y, Horie A (1984). Amyloid angiopathy and lobar cerebral haemorrhage. J Neurol, Neurosurg, and Psychiatry Vol 47, p 1203-1210

[73] Gatti L, Tinelli F, Scelzo E, et al. (2020). Understanding the pathophysiology of cerebral amyloid angiopathy. Int J Molec Sci Vol 21, p 3435-3455

Chapter 2

Diagnosis of Amyloidosis: From History to Current Tools

Richa Juneja, Prasad Dange and Rahul Arora

Abstract

The term amyloid encompasses a large variety of misfolded proteins with varying amino acids unified by the antiparallel beta-pleated sheet configuration and characteristic Congo red staining. The etiology of these proteins is equally varied, ranging from neoplastic plasma cell disorder, hereditary causes to inflammatory disorders. The protean clinical manifestation makes a high index of clinical suspicion the first crucial step in the diagnosis. A battery of investigations needs to be carried out for a complete diagnosis of amyloidosis and its underlying etiology. Biopsy with Congo red staining constitutes the most important modality for confirmation of amyloid. For further testing, varying modalities with increasing complexity, such as immunohistochemistry, electron microscopy, and mass spectrometry, need to be employed. We discuss, in the course of the current chapter, this fascinating protein from a clinical diagnosis perspective. The requisite investigations are also discussed in detail.

Keywords: amyloid, plasma cell, beta-pleated sheet, misfolded proteins, Congo red, mass spectrometry

1. Introduction

Amyloid is characterized by homogenous amorphous eosinophilic extracellular deposits in several tissues on routine histopathological examination. This amorphous proteinaceous substance is indeed very heterogeneous; however, all these types have some properties in common, which thereby define it as amyloid [1]. Understanding this core concept then makes it easy to understand the diagnostic approach for amyloid. Before proceeding with the diagnostic armamentarium available for amyloid, we briefly discuss various types of amyloid and their nomenclature.

2. Classification and nomenclature

Amyloid is characterized by some common properties as follows. These are fibrillary misfolded proteins that resist degradation by proteasome and macrophages leading to deposition. They can either be a normal protein with an inherent tendency to form amyloid when produced in excess (Example: ATTR) or result of genetic mutation giving rise to amyloidogenic protein. (Example: AApoAI) X-ray diffraction shows antiparallel ß-pleated sheet configuration noted on X-ray diffraction and Congo red stained section shows diagnostic apple-green birefringence

IntechOpen

under polarized light [2]. These properties bring them under one roof of amyloidosis. However, due to marked heterogeneity in chemical nature and therapeutic implications, amyloid is classified in several ways, as follows.

2.1 Systemic versus localized

Clinically, amyloid can be classified as systemic/generalized or localized based on whether it affects many organs/systems or affects only one site. Localized amyloid deposits are usually seen in the skin, larynx, and bladder. It is characterized by an indolent course requiring minimal intervention. However, recurrences can be a potential concern. At least 19 amyloid types are known to cause exclusive localized deposits. Systemic amyloidosis causes more generalized deposits, affecting the entire organ-like cardiac deposition in ATTR form or multisystem affection in AL amyloidosis. The systemic form is associated with 14 different forms of amyloidogenic proteins [3, 4]. Some forms like AL/AH/ATTR can cause localized deposits and more generalized systemic disease.

2.2 Primary versus secondary

Another popular way of classifying systemic amyloidosis is primary versus secondary amyloidosis. Primary is driven by clonal plasma cell proliferation, leading to excessive misfolded monoclonal light chain production, leading to fibril formation and amyloid deposition [5]. Whereas secondary amyloidosis is secondary to inflammatory processes like autoimmunity, infection likes tuberculosis.

Hereditary another distinct category is hereditary or familial amyloidosis where genetic mutation leads to the production of misfolded fibrillary protein (FAP).

We can also classify amyloidosis based on its biochemical nature. Thirty-six proteins have been identified as amyloidogenic in humans, and the list continues to grow with more types getting identified with sophisticated tests like mass spectrometry.

	Systemic/ localized/ both	Amyloid type	Precursor protein	Organ predominantly affected
Hereditary	Systemic	ATTR	Transthyretin, variants	PNS, ANS, heart, eye, leptomeninges
	Systemic	Aβ2M	β2 microglobulin, variants	ANS
	Systemic	AApoAI	Apolipoprotein A I, variants	Heart, liver, kidney, PNS, testis, larynx (C terminal variants), skin (C terminal variants)
	Systemic	AApoAII	Apolipoprotein A II, variants	Kidney
	Systemic	AApoCII	Apolipoprotein C II, variants	Kidney
	Systemic	AApoCIII	Apolipoprotein C III, variants	Kidney
	Systemic	AGel	Gelsolin, variants	Kidney, PNS, cornea
	Systemic	ALys	Lysozyme, variants	Kidney
	Systemic	AFib	Fibrinogen a, variants	Kidney
	Systemic	ACys	Cystatin C, variants	CNS, PNS, skin
	Systemic	ABri	ABriPP, variants	CNS

	Systemic/ localized/ both	Amyloid type	Precursor protein	Organ predominantly affected
	Localized	ADanb	ADanPP, variants	CNS
	Localized	Aβ	Aβ protein precursor, variant	CNS
	Localized	APrP	Prion protein, variant	CJD, GSS syndrome, fatal insomnia
	Systemic		Prion protein variant	PNS
Acquired	Both	AL	Immunoglobulin light chain	All organs, usually except CNS
	Both	AH	Immunoglobulin heavy chain	All organs except CNS
	Systemic	AA	(Apo) Serum amyloid A	All organs except CNS
	Systemic	ATTR	Transthyretin, wild type	Heart mainly in males, lung, ligaments, tenosynovium
	Systemic	Ab2M	β2-microglobulin, wild type	Musculoskeletal system
	Systemic	AApoAIV	Apolipoprotein A IV, wild type	Kidney medulla and systemic
	Systemic	ALECT2	Leukocyte chemotactic factor-2	Kidney primarily, Liver
	Localized	Aβ	Aβ protein precursor, wild type	CNS
	Localized	AaSyn	α-Synuclein	CNS
	Localized	ATau	Tau	CNS
	Localized	APrP	Prion protein, wild type	CJD, fatal insomnia
	Localized	ACal	(Pro)calcitonin	C-cell thyroid tumours
	Systemic	ACal	(Pro)calcitonin	Kidney
	Localized	AIAPP	Islet amyloid polypeptidec	Islets of Langerhans, insulinomas
	Localized	AANF	Atrial natriuretic factor	Cardiac atria
	Localized	APro	Prolactin	Pituitary prolactinomas, aging pituitary
	Localized	AIns	Insulin	Iatrogenic, local injection
	Localized	ASPCd	Lung surfactant protein	Lung
	Localized	ACor	Corneodesmosin	Cornified epithelia hair follicles
	Localized	AMed	Lactadherin	Senile aortic, media
	Localized	AKer	Kerato-epithelin	Cornea, hereditary
	Localized	ALac	Lactoferrin	Cornea
	Localized	AOAAP	Odontogenic ameloblast-associated protein	Odontogenic tumours
	Localized	ASem1	Semenogelin 1	Vesicula seminalis
	Localized	AEnf	Enfurvitide	Iatrogenic
	Localized	ACatKe	Cathepsin K	Tumour associated
	Localized	AEFEMP1e	EGF-containing fibulin-like extracellular matrix protein 1 (EFEMP1)	Portal veins Aging associated

Table 1.
This table summarizes the common amyloid proteins identified in humans with brief comments related to each of them [6].

2.3 Nomenclature

International society of amyloidosis (ISA) recommended in 2018 that the name of any amyloidosis start with A standing for amyloid followed by suffix suggestive of underlying pathogenic protein. Example- AH stands for the heavy chain of immunoglobulin giving rise to amyloid [6, 7]. However AH, AL are amyloid proteins, and AH amyloidosis is the disease.

For amyloidosis caused by various inherited mutations leading to fibrillary protein production, hereditary is the favored term compared to familial. In hereditary subset nomenclature recommendation by ISA says single letter coding for amino acid substitution can be used with mention of amino acid position where substitution is happening. Example: ATTRV30M or ALysI56T. To indicate the mutation is driving the amyloidosis, vATTR (variant) is recommended by ISA over (mutant) ATTRm (**Table 1**).

3. History of diagnostic tools for amyloid

3.1 Early advances: till the development of Congo red as a diagnostic tool

Like many other diseases, the first description of amyloid came from autopsy rooms. It evolved from classical gross description to gross staining with iodine and sulfuric acid, suggesting starch-like amyloid properties [8].

Botanist Matthias Schleiden followed by Rudolf Virchow used this term amyloid, and confusion about its starch-like nature continued [9, 10].

Initially, metachromatic stains were utilized to detect amyloid. However, later chemist Paul Böttiger discovered a textile dye named Congo red which can bind to amyloid and Puchtler described the method for histological preparation [11]. Since then Congo red staining and apple-green birefringence became the gold standard for establishing the amyloid diagnosis. This early history of diagnosis of amyloidosis is dealt with in better detail in another chapter of this book. Hence, we intend to focus on the history of evolving tools for amyloid typing.

3.2 Modern history of amyloid diagnosis-evolution of tools for amyloid typing

1959, Alan S Cohen and Calkin decoded the fibrillary nature of amyloid under the electron microscope [12].

Amyloid extraction followed by X-ray diffraction demonstrated cross beta-pleated sheet structure of amyloid by Eanes and Glenner [13].

More important application of amyloid extraction opened the door for understanding biochemical nature and hence the pathogenesis of different types of amyloid. Glenner and colleagues decoded that AL amyloid was indeed due to the light chain of immunoglobulin getting misfolded and producing amyloid. AL is the most common type of amyloidosis affecting humankind.

Identifying these different types of amyloid proteins is what is referred to as amyloid typing in today's diagnostic practices. As emphasized earlier this is the crucial part of work up as treatment may vary from bone marrow transplant for AL amyloidosis to liver transplant for others.

Amyloid typing tools exploit two principles; one is the immune platform where antibody against the antigen of interest (amyloid here) is allowed to react. The immune complex formed is detected by either fluorescence in immunofluorescence (IF), chromogen in immunohistochemistry (IHC), or coupled this immune reaction with electron microscopy localizing exact deposition of the complex in immuno-electron microscopy [14].

Among the above investigations, IHC and IF have the biggest advantage of being widely available today. However, over time, researchers found several limitations of these typing techniques like the IHC panel is usually limited to target AL, AA, and ATTR amyloid. These tests do not detect mutated and truncated forms and have cross-reactivity with non-amyloid proteins [15]. Immunofluorescence as a technique for amyloid typing needs frozen tissue and antibodies used lack specificity giving inconclusive results [16].

To overcome these shortcomings of immune methods for amyloid typing breakthrough technology of proteomics mass spectrometry was used. Vrana et al. used laser micro-dissection to extract the amyloid from Congo red positive bit of histopathology section and did a proteomic study with mass spectrometry to classify several types of amyloid by identifying the very nature of pathogenic protein giving rise to misfolded fibrils [17]. Modification of this technique is also developed for fat pad aspirate specimens. Details of these amyloid typing technologies will be discussed in the amyloid typing techniques section of this chapter.

Decoding the amyloid fibril to its true protein nature was possible with these typing tools. However, another aspect was to understand some types of amyloidosis that can be inherited and the treatment concerns they created.

Satoru Tawara and colleagues identified a point mutation in the gene coding for TTR mutant TTR-related FAP in 1983 [18]. To date, several hereditary types of amyloidosis have been identified, which are driven by various genetic events. Recent additions to this list have been fibrinogen A-α chain, lysozyme, apolipoprotein AII, and leucocyte chemotactic factor 2 [19].

This brings us to the end of a brief review of how the history of amyloid detection evolves from gross staining properties confusing it for starch to sophisticated tools understanding its true proteinaceous nature with typing of amyloid proteins and deciphering genetic events leading to a subset of these amyloid deposits. Knowing this background helps us to understand how we use these tools developed over decades and apply them today for the diagnostic workup of this rather unusual and mystifying disease.

4. Diagnostic approach to amyloidosis

4.1 Diagnosis starts by suspecting in clinic

Clinically it is relevant to first classify patients as having localized versus systemic amyloidosis. Localized amyloid is often only a cosmetic concern presenting as a nodule or a plaque most commonly in the skin. Localized cutaneous amyloid can be AD (keratin) depositing at the site of trauma or An Insulin at the site of injection, and many more. Rarely polyclonal plasma cells can give rise to a localized deposit of amyloidogenic light chain in skin, larynx, urinary bladder, and others. The localized form usually does not require extensive therapy, however, it can recur [3].

One of the challenges in establishing systemic amyloidosis diagnosis is suspecting it in the correct scenario and ordering the correct test. Coming across such patients should alert the treating physician to order broad screening tests for amyloid.

Patient may complain of nonspecific fatigue or weight loss, to symptoms and signs suggestive of the target organ involved. Classical presentations of systemic amyloidosis are nephrotic range proteinuria in renal amyloidosis, cardiac failure, sensorimotor and autonomic neuropathy without apparent cause [4].

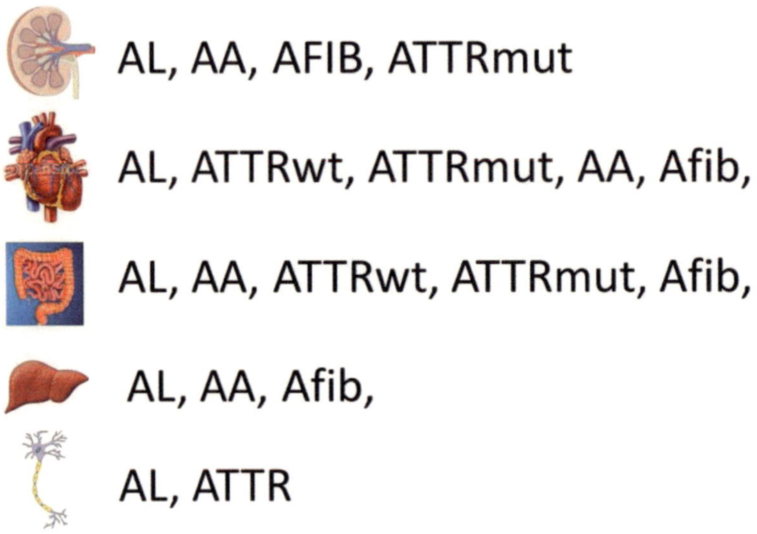

Figure 1.
Summary of the organ preference by various amyloidosis.

Primary amyloidosis (AL) is the most common type of systemic amyloidosis. The ratio of primary to non-primary is more skewed in America (20:1) than Europe (2:1), attributed to the common occurrence of hereditary familial Mediterranean fever in Europe. The kidney is the most common organ involved by all systemic amyloidosis except in ATTR. Other organs involved by AL type are the heart, liver kidney, and nervous system. Hepatomegaly with normal echotexture, easy bruising around eyes, and macroglossia are other classical pointers to amyloidosis, especially the commonest form, i.e. AL amyloidosis [3].

Several pointers in history help us to predict the type of amyloidosis. History of chronic inflammatory disease raises the possibility of secondary AA amyloid. Positive family history tilts the balance towards the genetic nature of illness initiating molecular testing for the same. The predominant organ involved also gives us the clue about the type of amyloidosis under investigation (**Figure 1**).

Based on history and clinical examination when suspicion for amyloid is a very high battery of lab tests are advised. **Table 2** gives a comprehensive list of lab tests to be ordered in a case of amyloid to establish the diagnosis with amyloid typing [20].

4.2 Imaging for amyloid diagnosis/non-invasive amyloid diagnosis

Imaging tools are indispensable when cardiac amyloidosis is suspected. In patients with left ventricular wall thickness > 12 mm and red flag signs like unexplained right-sided heart failure, proteinuria, ECG showing reduced QRS voltage and conduction defect, and disproportionately increased N-terminal pro B-type natriuretic peptide (NT-proBNP), one should suspect cardiac amyloidosis. More than 97% of cases of cardiac amyloidosis are primary AL type or transthyretin type (both wild and mutant) [21]. Recent position statement of the European Society of Cardiology Working Group on Myocardial and Pericardial Diseases proposed non-invasive diagnostic criteria for cardiac amyloidosis though it is applicable for ATTR type only. Other types of cardiac amyloidosis still require demonstration on Congo red positive birefringent deposits to establish their diagnosis, which is discussed later.

For establishing diagnosis and typing of amyloid
• Target organ or surrogate site (abdominal fat pad) biopsy
• H & E and Congo red stain
• IHC/Immunoelectron microscopy/ proteomic study for amyloid typing
• Serum protein electrophoresis (SPEP), Immunofixation electrophoresis (IFE), Serum free light chain assay (sFLC) for evidence of monoclonal plasma cell proliferation
• Bone marrow aspirate and biopsy with flowcytometry for clonal plasma cells
• Mutation studies for various hereditary amyloidosis
• Work up for rheumatoid arthritis, tuberculosis and other inflammatory conditions associated with AA amyloidosis
For confirming systemic involvement, assess distribution and complications
• Renal function test
• 24 hours urine protein/albumin
• Cardiac magnetic resonance/Echocardiography for cardiac involvement
• Pro NT-B-type natriuretic peptide
• ECG
• USG/ CT scan for liver span
• Alkaline phosphatase
• X ray or CT scan of lung
• GIT biopsy with evidence of amyloid
• SAP scintigraphy/technetium scintigraphy
• Coagulation screen

Table 2.
List of investigations in case of amyloidosis (adapted with permission from Juneja et al. [20]).

Echocardiography and cardiac MRI (CMR) are important imaging tools to establish cardiac amyloidosis diagnosis. Classical findings on Echocardiography have left ventricle thickness > 12 mm with two or more of the below

1. Grade 2 or worse diastolic dysfunction

2. Reduced tissue Doppler S′, E′, and A′ wave velocities (<5 cm/s)

3. Decreased LV global longitudinal strain (absolute value <−15%). Echocardiography findings have been recently given a scoring system to predict cardiac amyloidosis [22].

CMR shows diffuse sub-endocardial or transmural late gadolinium enhancement with abnormal gadolinium kinetics and/or extracellular volume ≥ 0.40%. These radiological findings need to be supported by either tissue evidence, i.e. endomyocardial or surrogate site biopsy showing Congo red positive deposits with amyloid typing for invasive diagnosis of cardiac amyloidosis.

However, for a second most common type of cardiac amyloidosis i.e. ATTR amyloidosis these Echocardiography and CMR findings can be supported with non-invasive radiotracer uptake base investigation like 99mTc-pyrophosphate (PYP) scintigraphy showing grade 2 or 3 myocardial radiotracer uptake and all three tests for monoclonal protein detection being negative [23]. The idea behind this approach is that these 3 tests namely serum protein electrophoresis, urine electrophoresis, immunofixation and serum-free light chain assay combined have>99%

sensitivity to pick up monoclonal protein [24]. These tests shall be discussed in more detail under amyloid typing as a test to demonstrate monoclonal protein detection. Negative results help us to exclude AL amyloidosis. High-grade tracer uptake with CMR/Echocardiography findings suggest the possibility of ATTR amyloidosis and pursue genetic testing to differentiate wild and mutant forms.

However, this again needs to be reemphasized that non-ATTR cardiac amyloidosis, any positivity for monoclonal protein, grade 1 scintigraphy results, and suspicious CMR/Echocardiography findings warrants invasive/tissue-based diagnosis of amyloid with amyloid typing which will be discussed in detail below and is applicable to different types of systemic amyloidosis.

4.3 Establish the tissue diagnosis of amyloidosis

4.3.1 Site of biopsy

When a clinical profile is highly suspicious of systemic amyloidosis, the first step in establishing the diagnosis is obtaining the tissue evidence of amyloid deposits.

Based on the complaints and lab findings, the organ involved can be targeted like liver or kidney. There is always a risk of bleeding, limited accessibility with these vital organs. However, for screening purposes either an abdominal fat pad or bone marrow can be targeted as it is involved in 80% of cases of systemic amyloidosis but may give a false negative result in ~15% cases [25].

4.3.2 Establishing the amyloid diagnosis on biopsy

Electron microscopy reveals the non-branching fibrillary nature of amyloid with a mean diameter of 10 nm (range 8 nm–12 nm). The fibrillary structure is not unique to amyloid as fibrils may be seen in other deposition diseases, such as immunotactoid glomerulonephritis and glomerular sclerosis. Electron microscopy shows differences in the characters of fibrils. However, we need a more widely available technique to confirm the deposits as amyloid [4].

Something as simple as routine histopathological evaluation of biopsy tissue with special stains comes to our rescue.

Amyloid is identified as an amorphous pink, homogenous, eosinophilic extracellular deposit on routine hematoxylin and eosin stain (**Figure 2a**). Though it has a classical appearance there are microscopic mimics. Fibrosis, Collagen, light chain and heavy chain deposits, and fibrin can potentially mimic amyloid; hence we need special stains to confirm amyloid [1].

As mentioned in detail in history, several stains enhance amyloid in different ways. Metachromatic stain to thioflavins showing fluorescence highlights amyloid. One stain that stood the test of time and is still most relevant to amyloid diagnosis is Congo red. X-ray diffraction revealed cross beta-pleated sheet structure of amyloid which potentially explains the mechanism of Congo red positivity and birefringence by amyloid.

The non-ionic hydrogen bond between amyloid and Congo red dye imparts it deep pink to red color. On polarization Congo red stained amyloid demonstrate apple-green birefringence, which is unique and diagnostic of amyloid unlike its mimics on histopathology (**Figure 2b** and **c**). Since then this text tile dye meant to stain cellulose fiber of fabric became an indispensable tool for amyloid diagnosis [11].

Congo red positivity with birefringence is now the part of the definition of amyloid. A routine light microscope can be easily converted to a polarizing microscope by adding a polarizer-analyzer pair in the light path [26]. However, one should remember that stain works better at alkaline PH on a thick cut section of 6 to 10 microns.

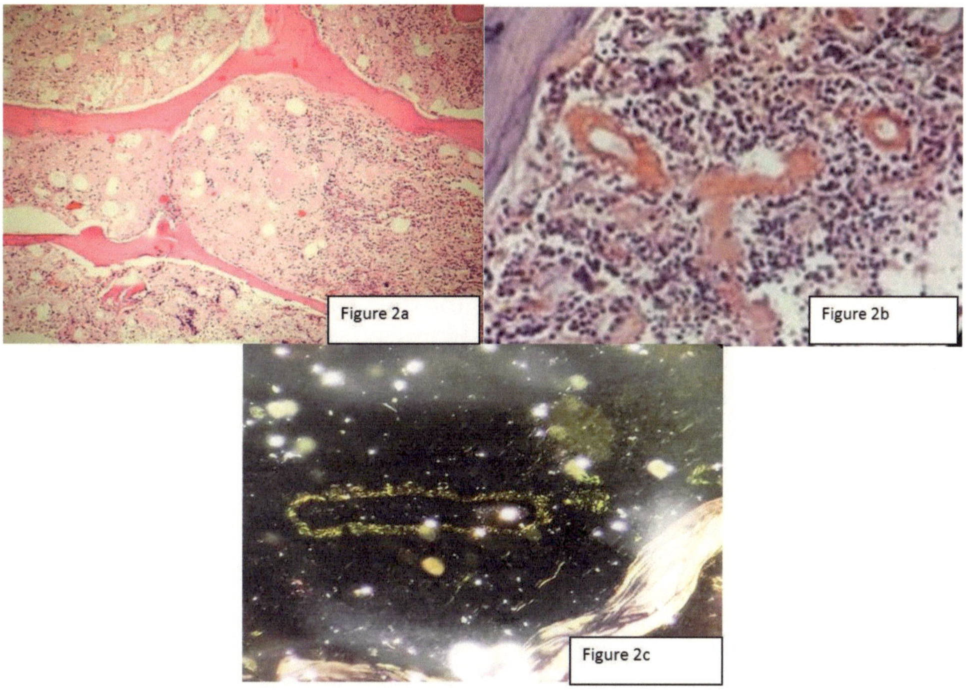

Figure 2.
a. H & E staining showing amorphous, extracellular, eosinophilic material (100X). b. Congo red stain showing deep pink to red-colored perivascular amyloid (400X). c. Amyloid deposits showing apple-green birefringence under polarized light (400X).

To conclude in the cases with high clinical suspicion one should order target organ or surrogate site biopsy and send for routine histopathological examination and special stain with Congo red. Documenting Congo red positive deposits with apple-green birefringence on polarization establishes the diagnosis of amyloidosis. It is also one of the diagnostic criteria for the most common systemic amyloidosis, i.e. primary AL amyloidosis by the International Myeloma Working group [27].

5. Subtyping of amyloid

5.1 Need of amyloid typing

While detection of amyloid is undoubtedly essential, equally important is to identify its subtype. Rather than being a separate disorder, amyloid deposition is often a manifestation of an underlying disease process. Amyloidosis causes symptoms based on organ involvement. However, some of the symptoms might be attributable to the underlying disease process independent of the amyloid deposition. Moreover, treatment of the underlying disorder is the only way to stop the progression of amyloid deposition. The therapy varies widely from liver transplant to bone marrow transplant depending on the type of amyloidosis. Sub-typing of the amyloid gives vital clues about the underlying disorder, highlighting the importance of identifying its subtype.

While apple-green birefringence in a Congo red section under the polarized microscope is sufficient for the detection of amyloid, its sub-typing is an uphill task.

Following issues need to be addressed after tissue diagnosis of amyloidosis is established.

a. Sub-typing of the amyloid.

b. Evaluate for the organs affected by amyloid deposits.

c. Evaluate for amyloid-independent symptoms attributable to the underlying cause.

d. Diagnose the underlying cause and formulate the best possible treatment option based on it.

Numerous techniques have evolved ranging from simple, widely available immunofluorescence to complicated scarcely available mass spectrometry to identify the subtype of amyloid. Each of these techniques has its own merits and will be discussed subsequently.

5.2 Tools of amyloid typing-immunofluorescence

Immunofluorescence (IF) is based on antigen–antibody reaction. The difference is that the antibody is tagged to a fluorescent substance necessitating a fluorescent microscope to visualize the reaction. The staining is done typically on frozen sections of unfixed tissue. Immunofluorescence can also be performed on formalin-fixed tissue (when fresh unfixed tissue is unavailable), albeit at a slightly lower sensitivity [28]. Since the fluorescence fades with time and exposure to light, it is necessary to view the slides immediately on staining and digitally archive them before it fades. Moreover, the repertoire of antibodies available for sub-typing by IF is limited.

Due to these numerous limitations, IF is not used for amyloid sub-typing. It is used to assess kidney and skin biopsies in which kappa or lambda staining may reveal restriction.

5.3 Immunohistochemistry

Immunohistochemistry (IHC) is a method that helps to detect and localize specific antigens in a tissue based on antigen–antibody reaction. In the current era, most of the IHC is being performed on formalin-fixed material for convenience and durability. The specific antibody against the antigen of interest is added to the tissue. After washing the unbound antibody, an enzyme (mostly horseradish peroxidase) tagged secondary antibody is added. This enzyme converts the chromogenic substance giving a colored reaction. When viewed under a microscope, the presence of the colored reaction product indicates the presence of the desired protein. Its location in relation to cell viz. extracellular, intra-nuclear, intra-cytoplasmic can also be determined [29].

The antibodies available to detect amyloid have increased steadily. Anti-amyloid P component antibody is used to detect the glycoprotein P that is associated with the amyloid deposits. It is independent of the type of amyloid and the anti-AP antibody is positive in virtually all the cases of amyloidosis [30]. Anti-kappa light chain, anti-lambda light chain, and anti-AA are the commonly used antibodies for amyloid sub-typing. Other antibodies include those directed against calcitonin, fibrinogen, lysozyme, transthyretin, β-2 microglobulin, and apolipoprotein A1.

The most significant advantage of IHC is the ease and convenience it offers in the diagnostic process. IHC for sub-typing is performed on the same tissue used for the detection of amyloid. No separate tissue processing needs to be done. Moreover, IHC is a widely available and routinely performed test. The slides can be easily photographed for digital archiving. The slides themselves can be preserved for a few years for review, if necessary. The diagnostic yield of immunohistochemistry is highly variable. While some centers have reported sensitivity and specificity nearing 90% [30, 31], others have reported being as low as 75% [32]. With correct standardization of the staining procedure, IHC is a very powerful and convenient tool for amyloid sub-typing.

However, IHC staining does come with some potential pitfalls that one needs to be aware of. In a large study including 169 biopsies, Anja et al. found that 13 biopsies could not be stained either due to insufficient tissue or failure of all the antibodies to stain the tissues [31]. The antibodies are typically manufactured using native protein as the antigen. Hence, in some cases with significant alteration in the protein structure during amyloidogenesis, the antibody may fail to stain the amyloid deposit leading to lower sensitivity [33]. The other important pitfall encountered by Anja et al. was non-specific staining in 51 cases. In these, the tissue showed positive staining with more than one antibody from among the panel of antibodies. In such cases, the antibody that stains strongly and homogeneously was considered positive while others were negative. However, in almost 33 cases the staining was inconclusive and clinical and other patient details had to be considered for final sub-classification. Intense staining with more than one antibody or inhomogeneous staining with 2 or more antibodies (in absence of strong staining by anyone antibody) are some of the pitfalls of immunohistochemistry. This inconclusive false-positive staining is either due to non-specific binding to non-amyloid protein or the presence of normal proteins within the amyloid deposits containing the epitope targeted by the antibody (e.g. plasma proteins entrapped in amyloid deposits may give false-positive reaction with anti-kappa and anti-lambda antibody). After thorough standardization of the procedure, a dedicated center may be able to reduce (but not eliminate) such inconsistencies.

In summary, due to easy availability, IHC is an excellent tool for sub-typing of the amyloid. However, both false positive and false negative staining reactions make it necessary to employ other diagnostic tools. A dedicated center with rigorous validation protocols for IHC may be able to achieve high sensitivity and specificity.

5.4 Immunoelectronmicroscope (IEC)

In principle, IEC is similar to IHC relying on the binding of a specific antibody to the amyloid. However, IEC does offer certain advantages over IHC that make it a very sensitive and specific modality for confirmation of the presence of amyloid and its sub-typing.

Transmission electron microscopy relies on a beam of electrons instead of light to visualize the tissue. The high-energy electrons make it possible to visualize the tissue at a much higher magnification without losing the resolution. Consequently, the processing of the tissue for electron microscopy differs vastly from processing for routine light microscopy. Fixative for electron microscopy is either glutaraldehyde or Karnovsky fixative (glutaraldehyde+formaldehyde). Though fresh tissue is preferred, formalin-fixed tissue can be re-processed for electron microscopy. The selected areas from semi-thin sections are further subjected to immunoelectron microscopy. The antigen–antibody reaction is visualized by using protein A/G gold conjugates. These gold conjugates appear as sharp electron-dense deposits [34].

The biggest advantage of IEC is the direct visualization of the amyloid fibrils. Thus, any non-specific binding of the gold-labeled antibody to non-amyloid proteins can be detected improving the specificity to more than 95%. Electron microscopy not only provides confirmatory detection of amyloid but immunostaining can also help in its sub-typing. In a large study involving 423 cases of systemic amyloidosis, the sensitivity of IEM was comparable to light microscopy (75–80%). The specificity in detection and sub-typing was however virtually 100% [35].

The limited availability of electron microscopes precludes its routine use. Also, the expertise needed for tissue processing and interpretation makes it out of most laboratories' reach. However, the use of IEM at a referral laboratory for the diagnosis of cases indeterminate on IHC is possible and may overcome the economic and technical constraints.

5.5 Mass spectrometry

Mass spectrometry is a powerful, modern tool for proteomics study. Proteomics, similar to genomics, is the study of all the proteins produced by an organism, an organ system, or an individual cell. Mass spectrometry uses a sophisticated multi-step process to isolate and identify the proteins by determining the molecular mass. Modern developments in mass spectrometry are towards devising ways to accurately quantify the various isolated proteins in the mixture [36].

The initial step is to isolate and concentrate the tissue of interest. In the context of amyloidosis, it involves careful separation of the congophilic amyloid deposits from the rest of the tissue. This is usually achieved through laser micro-dissection on a thick (6–8 micron) section of formalin-fixed tissue. The micro-dissected predominantly contains amyloid proteins along with other proteins. These proteins are extracted and then subjected to trypsin digestion to break them into fragments. The proteins need to be broken down to fragment peptides because intact proteins are too large to be analyzed efficiently by mass spectrometry. Once generated, these fragments are then separated from one another using high-performance liquid chromatography. These uncharged peptides cannot be subjected to mass spectrometry. The next step, probably the most significant, is imparting a charge to the peptides without dissociating or fragmenting them. Commonly done by electrospray ionization (ESI), the peptide can also be charged using matrix-assisted laser desorption/ionization (MALDI). These ionized peptides are then subjected to "flight" in an electromagnetic field. The movement of these peptides is dependent on their mass to charge ratio, the software analyses the data to determine the molecular mass. An expert interpretation is needed to make sense of the data and the software analysis to reach a definite conclusion about the various constituents of the protein mixture [37].

The detection and diagnosis of amyloidosis by MS relies on the detection of "amyloid signature" and detection of specific subtypes. Amyloid signature detects non-amyloid proteins that are universally associated with amyloid proteins irrespective of the amyloid subtype. Detection of these proteins gives proof of the presence of amyloid in the sample. These proteins are Serum Amyloid P component (SAP), apolipoprotein A4 (APOA4), and apolipoprotein E (APOE). Indeed, in a study by Vrana et al., 13 out of 20 Congo red negative subcutaneous fat aspirates showed the amyloid signature implying its higher sensitivity than conventional Congo red staining to detect amyloidosis [38]. Detection of a specific subtype depends on the detection of a specific protein. The sensitivity and specificity of MS for amyloid sub-typing are about 90% and nearly 100% respectively [39]. In some cases, the amyloid signature protein may be detected but sub-typing may not be possible by MS.

Apart from high sensitivity and specificity, the most significant utility is the identification of unknown and novel proteins. Unlike antibody-based methods (like IHC or IEM), MS characterizes all the protein in the micro-dissected material and hence rare cases of novel amyloid subtypes can also be diagnosed by MS. However, similar to IEM, high cost, necessary technical expertise makes MS out of reach for most laboratories.

6. Diagnosis of underlying disorder

Management of amyloidosis targets the underlying disorder. No definitive treatment can reverse the amyloid protein that is already deposited, and thus treatment aims to control the underlying disorder, preventing further amyloid deposition. Sub-typing of the amyloid is crucial for the diagnosis of the underlying disorder. Every effort to subtype the amyloid should be made. In case IHC is indeterminate, the sample is sent for immunoelectron microscopy or preferably mass spectroscopy to a referral lab. Once the amyloid is sub-typed, relevant testing can be performed to confirm the presence of the underlying disorder.

6.1 AL amyloid

AL amyloid is derived from the immunoglobulin light chain, either kappa or lambda. It is practically secondary to underlying plasma cell dyscrasia, rarely due to some other type of lymphoma. Plasma cell dyscrasias have been classified into different sub-types with specific diagnostic criteria [40]. Being a disorder that affects multiple systems, a battery of tests is needed for a detailed investigation of plasma cell dyscrasia. Amyloid deposition can be secondary to multiple myeloma or other monoclonal gammopathies like MGUS or asymptomatic myeloma. However, occasionally, it may occur in the absence of any detectable plasma cell dyscrasia in which case it is termed as Primary Amyloidosis. It must, however, be noted that even primary amyloidosis is due to an underlying clonal plasma cell proliferation that is so small that routine tests cannot detect it. In such cases, other investigations like urine electrophoresis and serum-free light chain assay may be helpful.

6.2 AA amyloid

AA amyloidosis is generally due to an underlying inflammatory condition such as chronic autoimmune diseases, including rheumatoid arthritis and inflammatory bowel disease, and chronic infections, like tuberculosis. Occasionally, familial Mediterranean fever may be the cause of AA amyloidosis. The cause of AA amyloid deposition is often dependent on the geography-inflammation associated with AA commoner in developing countries and familial Mediterranean fever is a commoner cause in people of the Mediterranean region especially Turks, non-Ashkenazi Jews, Arabs, and Armenians. Thus, in a case with AA amyloid deposits, the ethnicity of the patient along with a careful clinical examination of the patient will give a clue to the possible diagnosis. Further investigations in acquired amyloidosis will be directed towards identifying the underlying cause. In almost one-fifth of cases, the underlying cause may remain undiagnosed despite extensive investigations [41].

6.3 Hereditary amyloidosis

Diagnosis of hereditary disorders leading to amyloidosis hinges on the integration of information obtained by amyloid sub-typing, the clinical details of the patient, and the genetic test to detect the specific gene mutation.

6.4 Cases when amyloid sub-typing not possible

In occasional cases, despite best efforts, it may not be possible to subtype the amyloid on tissue biopsy. In such cases, identification of the underlying disease would be based on the clinical details and ancillary investigations. However, it must be noted that this approach may lead to misdiagnosis as more than one condition may co-exist. Most commonly, monoclonal gammopathy may co-exist with other causes of amyloidosis, especially the hereditary forms [42]. Some of the difficulties encountered in cases where amyloid typing is not possible on biopsy include:

1. Hereditary forms often present late in life and have variable penetrance making family history unreliable.

2. Monoclonal gammopathy is a common incidental finding in many elderly individuals. Its presence does not imply that the amyloid is AL type.

3. The pattern of organ involvement, though helpful, is often overlapping in many different types of amyloid.

Thus it is imperative that every effort must be made to subtype the amyloid on the biopsy material.

1. **Summary:** Amyloidosis is a disorder of deposition of misfolded protein in extracellular spaces. Heart, kidney, liver, blood vessels in various organs are principally affected organs. Chemically amyloid has vast heterogeneity, the common feature being misfolding of the abnormal protein to form beta-pleated sheets. The chemical heterogeneity stems from equally varying causes ranging from hereditary to acquired and malignant disorders.

The clinical manifestations usually pertain to the organ involved. Except for ATTR cardiac amyloidosis, tissue biopsy is crucial for confirmation and chemical sub-typing of amyloid. Characteristic apple-green birefringence under polarized light is a Congo red stained tissue is still the most widely used technique for amyloid detection. IHC, immune-electron microscopy, and mass spectrometry are increasingly complex but efficient tools for chemical sub-typing of the amyloid. Apart from that, a battery of investigations is required for confirmation of underlying disorder and to assess the organs involved by amyloid. Diagnosis of amyloidosis starts from suspicion in the clinic. Following algorithm summarizes the diagnostic approach for a suspected case of amyloidosis.

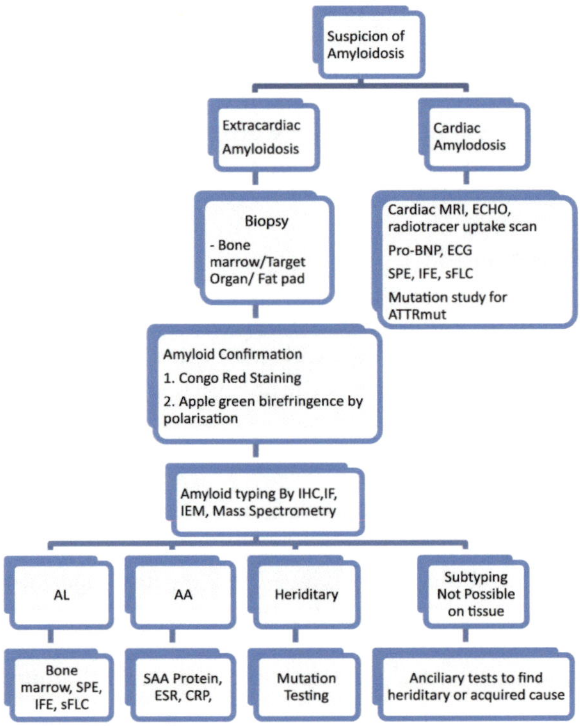

7. Conclusions

Science has evolved, and there has been significant improvement in our understanding of this complex disease called amyloidosis. This has led to better diagnostic tools, therapeutic options, and eventually better care for patients suffering from this group of illnesses. However, we still strive to develop techniques for early detection, preventive strategies, and curative options for this mysterious disease.

Conflict of interest

Nil.

Author details

Richa Juneja[1*], Prasad Dange[2] and Rahul Arora[3]

1 All India Institute of Medical Sciences, Nagpur, India

2 All India Institute of Medical Sciences, Raipur, India

3 HCG—NCHRI, Nagpur, India

*Address all correspondence to: drrichajuneja@gmail.com

References

[1] Kumar V, Abbas AK, Aster JC, Perkins JA. Robbins Basic Pathology. 10th ed. Philadelphia, Pennsylvania: Elsevier; 2018

[2] Picken MM. The pathology of amyloidosis in classification: A review. Acta Haematologica. 2020;**143**(4):322-334

[3] Leung N, Nasr SH, Sethi S. How I treat amyloidosis: The importance of accurate diagnosis and amyloid typing. Blood. 2012;**120**(16):3206-3213

[4] Mollee P, Renaut P, Gottlieb D, Goodman H. How to diagnose amyloidosis. Internal Medicine Journal. 2014;**44**(1):7-17

[5] Gertz MA. The classification and typing of amyloid deposits. American Journal of Clinical Pathology. 2004;**121**(6):787-789

[6] Benson MD, Buxbaum JN, Eisenberg DS, Merlini G, Saraiva MJM, Sekijima Y, et al. Amyloid nomenclature 2018: Recommendations by the International Society of Amyloidosis (ISA) nomenclature committee. Amyloid. 2018;**25**(4):215-219

[7] Benson MD, Buxbaum JN, Eisenberg DS, Merlini G, Saraiva MJM, Sekijima Y, et al. Amyloid nomenclature 2020: Update and recommendations by the International Society of Amyloidosis (ISA) nomenclature committee. Amyloid. 2020;**27**(4):217-222

[8] Kyle RA. Amyloidosis: A convoluted story: Historical review. British Journal of Haematology. 2001;**114**(3):529-538

[9] Tanskanen M. "Amyloid" — Historical Aspects. Rijeka: InTech; 2013

[10] Sipe JD, Cohen AS. Review: History of the amyloid fibril. Journal of Structural Biology. 2000;**130**(2): 88-98

[11] Puchtler H, Sweat F, Levine M. On the binding of congo red by amyloid. The Journal of Histochemistry and Cytochemistry. 1962;**10**(3):355-364

[12] Cohen AS, Calkins E. The isolation of amyloid fibrils and a study of the effect of collagenase and hyaluronidase. The Journal of Cell Biology. 1964;**21**: 481-486

[13] Sunde M, Blake C. The Structure of Amyloid Fibrils by Electron Microscopy and X-Ray Diffraction. Advances in Protein Chemistry. Newyork: Elsevier; 1997. pp. 123-159

[14] Dasari S, Theis JD, Vrana JA, Rech KL, Dao LN, Howard MT, et al. amyloid typing by mass spectrometry in clinical practice: A comprehensive review of 16,175 samples. Mayo Clinic Proceedings. 2020;**95**(9):1852-1864

[15] Solomon A, Murphy CL, Westermark P. Unreliability of immunohistochemistry for typing amyloid deposits. Archives of Pathology & Laboratory Medicine. 2008;**132**(1):14 author reply 14-5

[16] Satoskar AA, Burdge K, Cowden DJ, Nadasdy GM, Hebert LA, Nadasdy T. Typing of amyloidosis in renal biopsies: Diagnostic pitfalls. Archives of Pathology & Laboratory Medicine. 2007;**131**(6):917-922

[17] Vrana JA, Gamez JD, Madden BJ, Theis JD, Bergen HR 3rd, Dogan A. Classification of amyloidosis by laser microdissection and mass spectrometry-based proteomic analysis in clinical biopsy specimens. Blood. 2009;**114**(24): 4957-4959

[18] Tawara S, Nakazato M, Kangawa K, Matsuo H, Araki S. Identification of

amyloid prealbumin variant in familial amyloidotic polyneuropathy (Japanese type). Biochemical and Biophysical Research Communications. 1983;**116**(3): 880-888

[19] Benson MD, James S, Scott K, Liepnieks JJ, Kluve-Beckerman B. Leukocyte chemotactic factor 2: A novel renal amyloid protein. Kidney International. 2008;**74**(2):218-222

[20] Juneja R, Pati HP. Approach to the diagnosis of amyloidosis. Indian Journal of Hematology and Blood Transfusion. 2020;**36**(2):246-253

[21] Garcia-Pavia P, Rapezzi C, Adler Y, Arad M, Basso C, Brucato A, et al. Diagnosis and treatment of cardiac amyloidosis. A position statement of the European Society of Cardiology Working Group on Myocardial and Pericardial Diseases. European Journal of Heart Failure. 2021;**23**(4):512-526

[22] Boldrini M, Cappelli F, Chacko L, Restrepo-Cordoba MA, Lopez-Sainz A, Giannoni A, et al. Multiparametric echocardiography scores for the diagnosis of cardiac amyloidosis. JACC: Cardiovascular Imaging. 2020;**13**(4): 909-920

[23] Gillmore JD, Maurer MS, Falk RH, Merlini G, Damy T, Dispenzieri A, et al. Nonbiopsy Diagnosis of cardiac transthyretin amyloidosis. Circulation. 2016;**133**(24):2404-2412

[24] Palladini G, Russo P, Bosoni T, Verga L, Sarais G, Lavatelli F, et al. Identification of amyloidogenic light chains requires the combination of serum-free light chain assay with immunofixation of serum and urine. Clinical Chemistry. 2009;**55**(3): 499-504

[25] Gertz MA. Immunoglobulin light chain amyloidosis: 2016 update on diagnosis, prognosis, and treatment. American Journal of Hematology. 2016;**91**(9):947-956

[26] Anil DP, Sudhir DP, Saksena A, Khurana N. An affordable, indigenous polarizer-analyser system with inbuilt retardation plate function to detect birefringence using 3d glasses: An experience. Journal of Clinical and Diagnostic Research. 2016;**10**(1): EC12-EC14

[27] Rajkumar SV, Dimopoulos MA, Palumbo A, Blade J, Merlini G, Mateos M-V, et al. International Myeloma Working Group updated criteria for the diagnosis of multiple myeloma. The Lancet Oncology. 2014;**15**(12):e538-e548

[28] Valencia-Guerrero A, Deng A, Dresser K, Bouliane G, Cornejo KM. The value of direct immunofluorescence on proteinase-digested formalin-fixed paraffin-embedded skin biopsies. The American Journal of Dermatopathology. 2018;**40**(2):111-117

[29] Taylor CR, Shi SR, Barr NJ. Techniques of Immunohistochemistry: Principles, Pitfalls and Standardization. In: Dabbs DJ, editor. Diagnostic Immunohistochemistry. 3rd ed. Philadelphia: Elsevier publications; 2010. pp. 1-41

[30] Schönland SO, Hegenbart U, Bochtler T, Mangatter A, Hansberg M, Ho AD, et al. Immunohistochemistry in the classification of systemic forms of amyloidosis: A systematic investigation of 117 patients. Blood. 2012;**119**(2): 488-493

[31] Kebbel A, Röcken C. Immunohistochemical classification of amyloid in surgical pathology revisited. The American Journal of Surgical Pathology. 2006;**30**(6):673-683

[32] Gilbertson JA, Theis JD, Vrana JA, Lachmann H, Wechalekar A, Whelan C, et al. A comparison of immunohistochemistry and mass spectrometry for determining the

amyloid fibril protein from formalin-fixed biopsy tissue. Journal of Clinical Pathology. 2015;**68**(4):314-317

[33] Wisniowski B, Wechalekar A. Confirming the Diagnosis of Amyloidosis. Acta Haematologica. 2020;**143**(4):312-321

[34] Donini U, Casanova S, Zucchelli P, Linke RP. Immunoelectron microscopic classification of amyloid in renal biopsies. The Journal of Histochemistry and Cytochemistry. 1989;**37**(7):1101-1106

[35] Fernández de Larrea C, Verga L, Morbini P, Klersy C, Lavatelli F, Foli A, et al. A practical approach to the diagnosis of systemic amyloidoses. Blood. 2015;**125**(14):2239-2244

[36] Bantscheff M, Schirle M, Sweetman G, Rick J, Kuster B. Quantitative mass spectrometry in proteomics: A critical review. Analytical and Bioanalytical Chemistry. 2007;**389**(4):1017-1031

[37] Picken MM. Proteomics and mass spectrometry in the diagnosis of renal amyloidosis. Clinical Kidney Journal. 2015;**8**(6):665-672

[38] Vrana JA, Theis JD, Dasari S, Mereuta OM, Dispenzieri A, Zeldenrust SR, et al. Clinical diagnosis and typing of systemic amyloidosis in subcutaneous fat aspirates by mass spectrometry-based proteomics. Haematologica. 2014;**99**(7):1239-1247

[39] Abildgaard N, Rojek AM, Møller HE, Palstrøm NB, Nyvold CG, Rasmussen LM, et al. Immunoelectron microscopy and mass spectrometry for classification of amyloid deposits. Amyloid. 2020;**27**(1):59-66

[40] Rajkumar SV. Updated diagnostic criteria and staging system for multiple myeloma. American Society of Clinical Oncology Educational Book. 2016;**35**:e418-e423

[41] Lane T, Pinney JH, Gilbertson JA, Hutt DF, Rowczenio DM, Mahmood S, et al. Changing epidemiology of AA amyloidosis: Clinical observations over 25 years at a single national referral centre. Amyloid. 2017;**24**(3):162-166

[42] Lachmann HJ, Booth DR, Booth SE, Bybee A, Gilbertson JA, Gillmore JD, et al. Misdiagnosis of hereditary amyloidosis as AL (primary) amyloidosis. The New England Journal of Medicine. 2002;**346**(23):1786-1791

Chapter 3

Therapeutic Approaches for Alzheimer's Disease: New Perspectives

Ivo Ilvan Kerppers, Andressa Panegalli Hosni, Andressa Leticia Miri, Maria Elvira Ribeiro Cordeiro, Flávio Klinpovous Kerppers, Mariane Maria Silveira Vieira de Lima, Ana Carolina Dorigoni Bini, Felipe Figueiredo Moreira, Patricia Pacheco Tyski Suckow, Eliane Gonçalves de Jesus Fonseca, Larissa Sakis Bernardi and Paulo Renato de Oliveira

Abstract

Alzheimer's disease (AD) was defined as a neurodegenerative disorder, being more affected in the elderly. It is estimated that every 3.2 seconds a person in the world is affected by the high disease that rate in 2050 to 1 second. Therefore, research has been carried out on new therapeutic approaches, such as Transcranial Photobiomodulation and treatment based on antioxidants, such as Resveratrol. Therefore, the objective is to conduct a literature review on these two approaches and their effects on the treatment of AD. It was carried out according to the PRISMA recommendation and the articles were selected according to the years of publication (between 2015 and 2020) and extracted from the following databases: Science Direct, PubMed PMC, Scopus, PubMed NCBI, SciELO, LILACS, MEDLINE and PEDro. In several studies it has been reported that both therapies provide improvements at the molecular and behavioral level, recovering brain functions, acting in a neuroprotective way, improving quality of life, with few adverse effects and in a less invasive way. Thus, both treatments have numerous benefits that can be useful in the treatment of AD. However, there is a need for further research that includes interventions with greater specificity and control, so that they are defined as ideal doses and treatment protocols.

Keywords: Alzheimer's disease, dementia, photobiomodulation, LED, resveratrol, β-amyloid

1. Introduction

Over the past few years Alzheimer's disease (AD) has been studied as a designation of neurodegenerative dysfunction, leading to the most causal dementia in the elderly population [1]. According to the International Alzheimer's Association

(2015), it is estimated that there are approximately 46.8 million people with dementia in the world, and it is believed that this number will double every 20 years, reaching 74.7 million in 2030 and to 131.5 million in 2050. Therefore, it is calculated that every 3.2 seconds, a new case of dementia is detected in the world and a prediction for 2050 is a new case every second [2].

Alzheimer's disease (AD) is characterized by several factors, such as the loss of cholinergic neurons, the formation of intracellular fibrillar tangles of the hyperphosphorylated tau proteins, and due to the abnormal processing of amyloid precursor proteins that causes extracellular deposition of βA proteins [3, 4]. Therefore, it is known as a progressive neurodegenerative disorder that is related to the individual's age and causes gradual physical and mental decline resulting in death [5, 6].

Memory impairment is not always the main symptom presented in patients with Alzheimer's disease [7]. Some patients may experience significant disturbances in the visuospatial or language functions [8].

2. Amyloid cascade hypothesis

This hypothesis suggests that the characteristic neurodegeneration of AD occurs due to the accumulation of beta-amyloid (βA) protein in several brain areas, triggering the formation of senile plaques and a series of neuron injuries related processes, and formation of neurofibrillary clusters of the tau protein, which lead to neuronal dysfunction and cell death (**Figure 1**) [10–12].

The deposition of senile plaques is a result of an abnormal processing of amyloid β protein, induced by errors in the proteolytic cleavage of amyloid precursor protein by β and γ secretases. This process results in the production of different fragments, which are: the β amyloid protein 1–42, highly neurotoxic and prone to aggregation, found in the brains of patients with AD; β amyloid 1–40, a soluble and less neurotoxic protein that contributes to local plasticity and is found in healthy brains; and the β amyloid protein 1–43, presenting high amyloidogenic and neurotoxic potential, capable of depositing before the other fragments. In AD patients, the proportion of neurotoxic forms is significantly higher than β 1–40 amyloid [10–12]

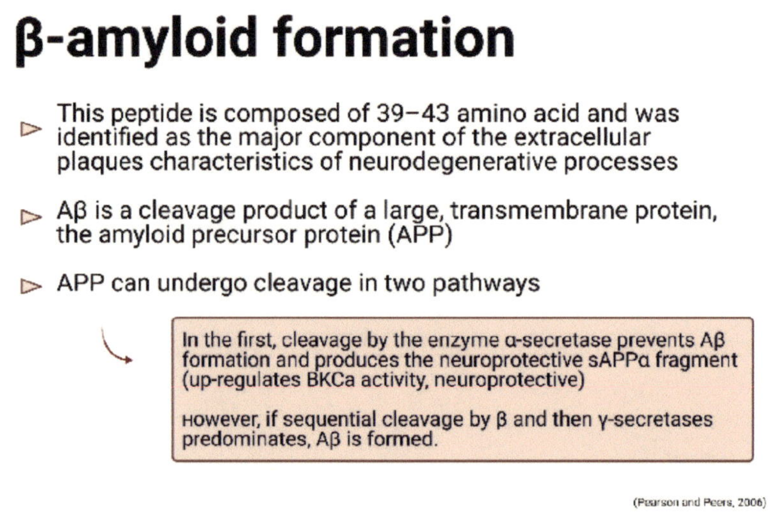

Figure 1.
β-amyloid (βA) formation [9]. Source: personal file.

Thus, the excess of βA- protein formed in the brain can trigger the formation of senile plaques, lead to inflammation, oxidative stress, hyperphosphorylation of the tau protein and, consequently, cause dementia (**Figure 2**) [10–12].

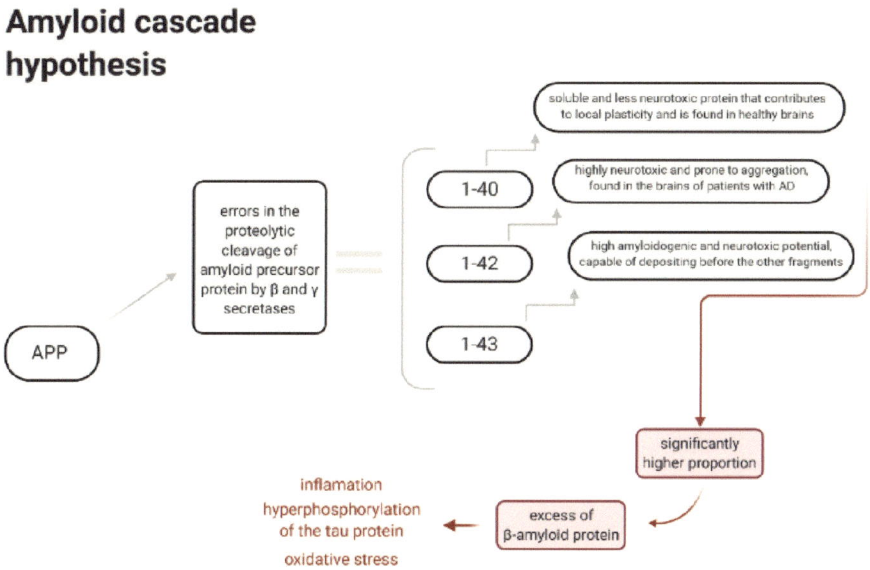

Figure 2.
Simplified schematic of the amyloid cascade. Source: Personal file.

3. Tau protein

The Tau protein is strongly associated to the responsibility of stabilizing and connecting the microtubes of the axions and dendrites. Conformational modifications in these structures and the accumulation of amyloid fragments appear to be responsible for the hyperphosphorylation of the tau protein (**Figure 3**) [14].

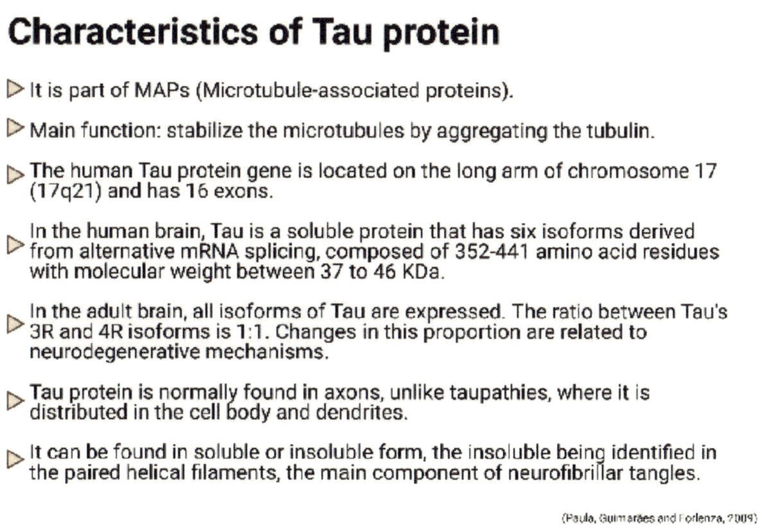

Figure 3.
Characteristics of tau protein [13]. Source: Personal file.

The hyperphosphorylation of tau in AD begins primarily in the intracellular process with the sequestration of regular tau and other proteins associated to the microtubes, causing a structural failure and thus compromising the neuronal and synaptic function [15].

The hyperphosphorylation hypothesis is due to the fact that, after the phosphorylation, an insoluble filamentous product is generated, which possibly causes the deregulation of the cytoplasmic cascade of phosphorylation and dephosphorylations. There is also a relation that the aggregations of β-amyloid may be the activating event of the protein hyperphosphorylation (**Figure 4**).

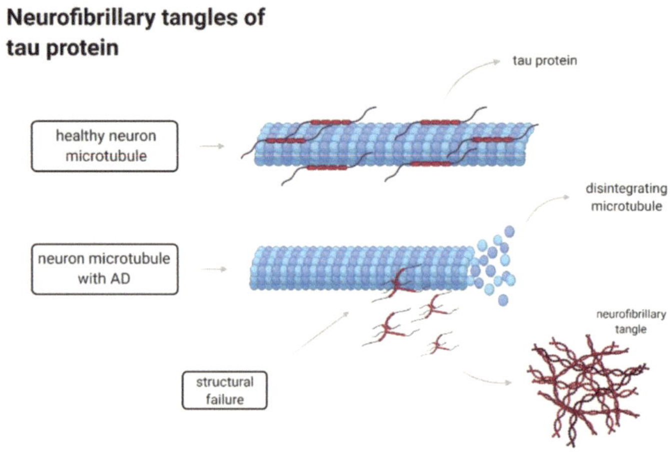

Figure 4.
Representation of the structural failure of neuronal microtubules and formation of tau protein tangles. Source: Personal file.

4. Metal hypothesis

The metal hypothesis is based on the precipitation of β-amyloid by zinc and copper radicalization, ionic zinc and copper are capable of accelerating the aggregation of Aβ, the main component of the deposition of β-amyloid [16, 17]. This hypothesis is related to the disturbance of endogenous metals in the brain, the ionic zinc and copper probably act on the cortical glutamatergic synapse, modulating the response of the inotropic receptor activated by the glutamic acid (NMDA), which can explain the vulnerability of β-amyloid to the abnormal interaction with the metallic ions on the synaptic region, leading to the aggregation and causing toxicity

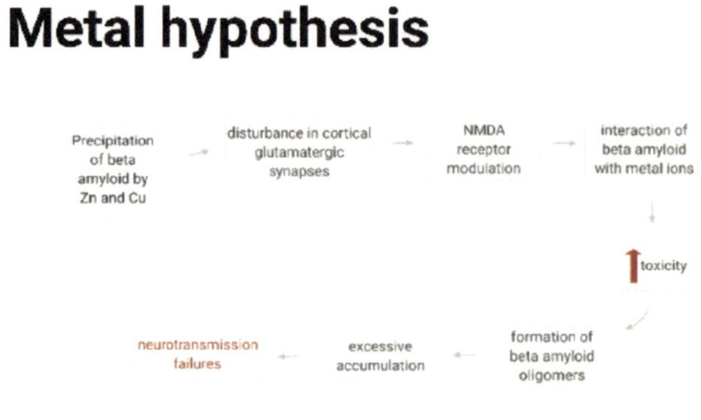

Figure 5.
Simplified scheme of the metal hypothesis. Source: Personal file.

[16]. The metals in the synapses can also lead to the formation of Aβ oligomers that have the role of modulating the long-term potentiation, which controls synaptic levels of the NMDA receptor, and this excessive accumulation of Aβ oligomers on the synaptic cleft affect the synaptic neurotransmission (**Figure 5**) [17].

5. Oligomeric hypothesis

The βA is one of the main mechanisms associated to Alzheimer's disease, and it has two main alloforms, Aβ 1–40 and Aβ 1–42, the last with more toxic oligomers [18, 19]. Studies show that the soluble oligomers, unlike the plaques, are the main cause of the synaptic disfunction and neurodegeneration. Oligomeric soluble Aβ interacts with several proteins, such as NMDA glutamatergic receptors and some proteins responsible for the maintenance of glutamate homeostasis, such as absorption and liberation [18].

It was discovered that βA oligomers were seen as intermediates in the path of disease-causing fibrils instead of impelling fully developed conditions. After that, oligomers were reported as a possible cause of Alzheimer's disease and neuronal death [20].

In the 2000s it was possible to understand that the βA fibrils are weakly toxic, but induce the neuroinflammation and, when agglomerating, they become dense and tend to detach and turn into oligomers. It is believed that currently βA oligomers exert their harmful effects connecting directly to the neuron membranes or to other specific receptors such as the insulin and glutamate (NMDA) ones, which are necessary for the neuronal signaling (**Figure 6**) [20].

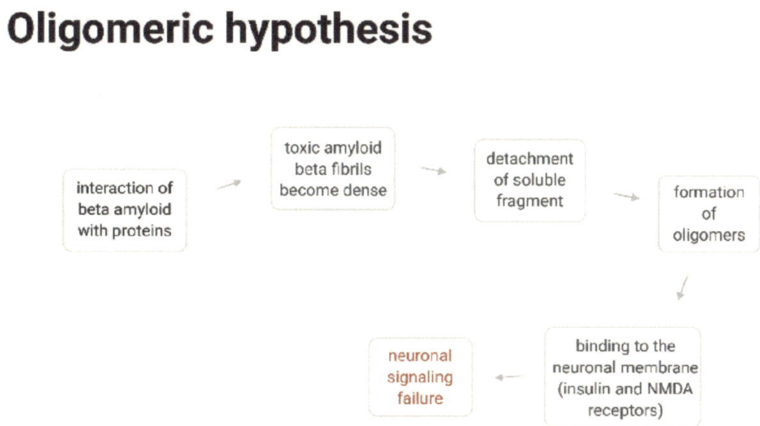

Figure 6.
Simplified scheme of the oligomeric hypothesis. Source: Personal file.

6. Glutamatergic dysfunction

The glutamatergic hypothesis refers to the biggest excitatory system of the central nervous system, the glutamatergic system. In AD, as well as in other acute and chronic neurodegenerative diseases, the loss of neurons may be due to an excessive synaptic excitation mediated by the glutamate amino acid, which explains the other denomination of the hypothesis as excito-toxic [11].

The glutamatergic system includes ionotropic and metabotropic receptors, both activated by glutamate, but in this hypothesis the ionotropic receptors stand out, such as NMDA, α-amino-3-hidroxi-5-metil-4-isoxazolepropionic acid (AMPA) and kainate, which contain ionic channels related to the neuronal polarization and depolarization processes [11, 21].

The NMDA receptors are responsible for the control of ion conductance, and when activated they determine mainly the entrance of Ca^{+2}, which increases the intensity and duration of the depolarization of the post-synaptic neuron, characterizing the long-term potentiation (LTP), which strengthens and shapes synapses, influencing phenomena such as learning and memory [11].

The activation of these receptors is essential, but in excess it can create pathogenic mechanisms related to neurodegenerative processes due to the calcium homeostasis, for when it is in high amounts in the intercellular medium, it can operate in the process of neuron degeneration and death (**Figure** 7) [21].

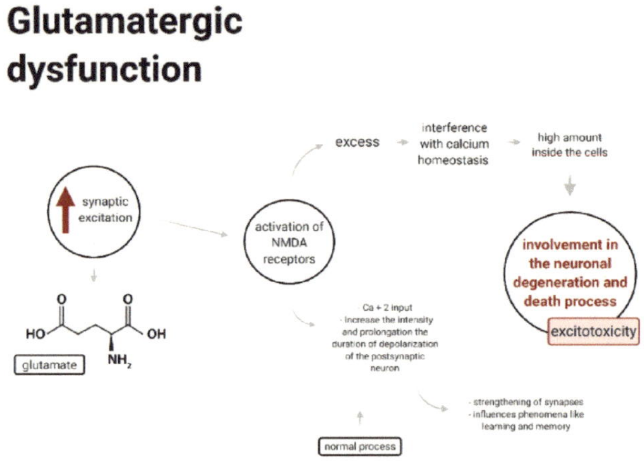

Figure 7.
Simplified scheme of the hypothesis of glutamatergic dysfunction. Source: Personal file.

7. Cholinergic hypothesis

The importance of acetylcholine (ACh) in the learning process and memory is known since the 70's, when studies showed a reduction of choline acetyltransferase (enzyme that synthesizes ACh) in the cortex and hippocampus, and less cholinergic neurons on Meynert's basal nucleus in subjects with AD [11, 22].

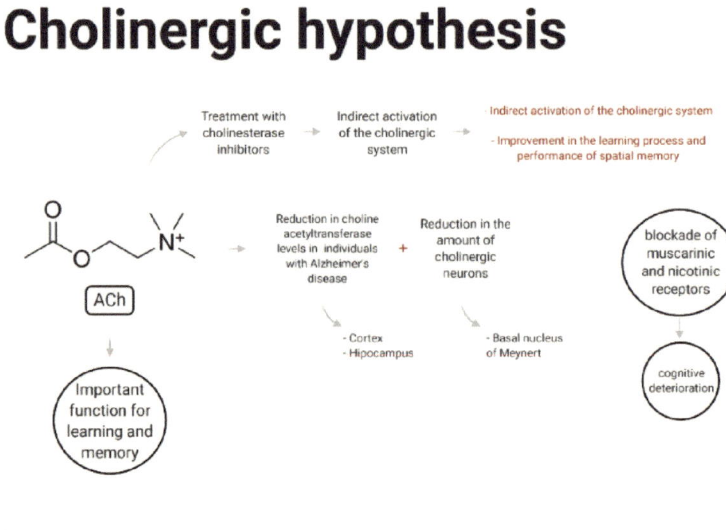

Figure 8.
Simplified scheme of the cholinergic hypothesis. Source: Personal file.

It was demonstrated that substances that inhibit acetylcholinesterase (enzyme that degrades ACh) cause positive effects on the learning and spatial learning performance, due to an indirect activation of the cholinergic system [22].

In addition to that, it is been reported that the blocking of muscarinic and nicotinic receptors leads to cognitive deterioration, indicating the importance of two kinds of receptors in the mechanism of memory and learning (**Figure 8**) [23].

8. Type 3 diabetes hypothesis

Metabolically, the brain is one of the most active organs of the human body because it processes big amounts of carbohydrates to generate energy as ATP. The brain does not count with the possibility of turning different substrates into energy, therefore, there is a higher use of glucose, and in the event that this supply or the ability of metabolization are compromised, this organ tends to become unprotected, and synapses failures are likely to happen, resulting in cognitive alterations [24].

Insulin has an important role in memory processing, it is capable of crossing the hematoencephalic barrier and is also produced in the brain tissue. Patients with AD show reduced insulin concentration and a smaller number of its receptors. When this is corrected with pharmacological intervention, there is an improvement in the processes related to cognition [25].

Also, studies show that toxic effects of βA might cause resistance to insulin, and this process may lead to an accumulation of βA, which constitutes in a positive feedback associated to the progressive neurodegeneration process characteristic of AD (**Figure 9**) [25, 26].

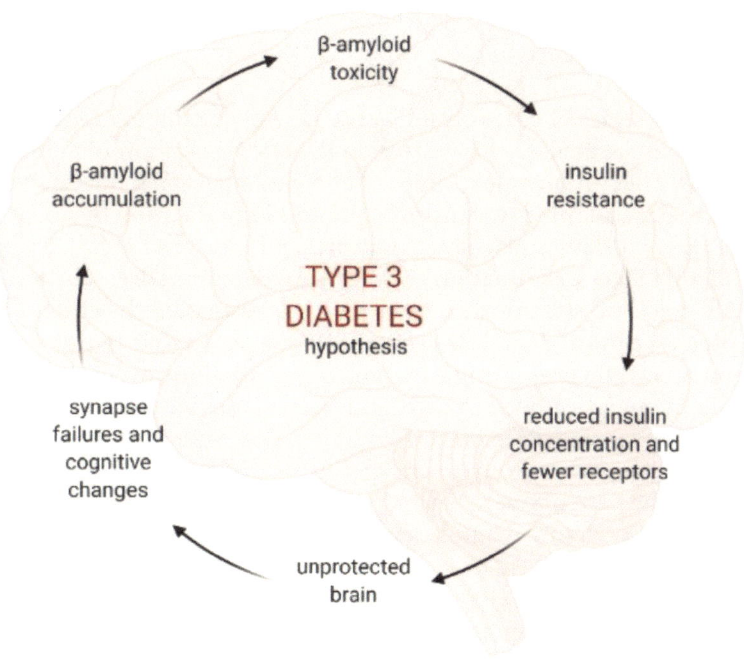

Figure 9.
Simplified scheme of the type 3 diabetes hypothesis. Source: Personal file.

9. New therapeutic approaches

Because there are only two classes of compounds commercially available for the AD treatment, and due to the failure of other approaches, several studies have been carried out in search of new therapies that are equally effective, safe, or better for treating the disease [10]. In this chapter, two forms of therapies that have been widely studied are discussed, namely: transcranial photobiomodulation (with LED) and treatment with antioxidants (Resveratrol).

9.1 Research method and inclusion of articles

The evaluation of clinical trials carried out on models of Alzheimer's and/or dementia that were treated by Photobiomodulation using light emitting diodes (LEDs) and Resveratrol was performed.

It was carried out in accordance with the PRISMA recommendation, which consists of a checklist with 27 items and a flowchart in four stages that assist in the eligibility of the selected questionnaires and work development.

For the Transcranial Photobiomodulation approach, academic articles published between 2015 and 2020 will be selected in the following databases: Science Direct, PubMed PMC, Scopus, PubMed NCBI, SciELO, LILACS, MEDLINE e PEDro. The descriptors will be in the English language only: Alzheimer's disease, light-emitting diode.

For treatments with Resveratrol, articles published between 2015 and 2020 will be selected and found in the following databases: Science Direct, PubMed PMC, Scopus, PubMed NCBI, SciELO, LILACS e MEDLINE. The descriptors will be in English: Resveratrol, Alzheimer's, neuroprotection.

Eight and six articles were selected to Transcranial Photobiomodulation and Resveratrol, respectively, to elaborate the discussion of this work.

9.2 Description of articles

9.2.1 Transcranial photobiomodulation (using LED)

In a report of a series of cases on subjects with AD or mild to moderately severe dementia, Saltmarche et al. [27] investigated the effects of photobiomodulation by 810 nm LED. The sample was composed of 5 patients with moderate to severe AD. The therapeutic adopted was infrared photo-biomodulation by pulsed LED (810 nm, 10 Hz), the device placed transcranial and intranasally for 12 weeks. Were used Mini Mental State Examination (MMSE), Alzheimer's Disease Assessment Scale (ADAS- cog) and statistical analysis, being investigated the effect of photo-biomodulation on clinical dementia. The results suggested that significant improvement in dementia while presenting functional increase, improvement of sleep, and less outbreaks of anxiety as well as rage, and that this device can be used safely and that there were no adverse effects.

Chao [28] used 8 participants (mean age: 79.8 ± 5.8 years old) diagnosed with dementia. The patients were treated with intranasally photobiomodulation with the Vielight Neuro Gamma device three times a week for 12 weeks and analyzed by Alzheimer Disease Assessment Scale-cognitive subscale (ADAS-cog); Neuropsychiatric Inventory (NPI); Magnetic resonance. The results were based on cognitive and behavioral function, cerebral perfusion, and functional connectivity at rest. It was found that the therapy provided improvements in ADAS-cog and PNI, increased cerebral perfusion and the enhancement of the connectivity between the posterior cingulate cortex and the lateral parietal nodes in the network in a standard way. Furthermore, the therapy was well tolerated and not associated with any adverse effects, indicating potential use as a viable home treatment for patients with dementia and AD.

Purushothuman et al. [29] used 2 models of mice with AD, a tau model K369I (K3), containing 15 animals and the other βA model APPs/PSEN1dE9 (APP-PS1) containing 18 animals. The therapeutic adopted was light from the LED device (670 nm), cycles of 90s (4 J/cm^2), 5 days a week, for 4 weeks, exposed 1 to 2 cm above the head. In relation the methods of analysis, they used histology by the Bielschowsky silver staining method, morphological analysis, histochemical analysis, and statistical analysis. Evaluating the effects on the cerebellar region, was observed that the positive effects of LED extend to the other brain regions; provoking a reduction of the neurodegenerative effects caused by AD in the cerebellum, such as the deposition of βA, neurofibrillary tangle formation and oxidative stress damage. So, in the findings of Purushothuman, LED was shown as an effective and safe alternative for treatment of neurodegenerative effects, being able to minimize and delay the pathological changes caused by dementia in different regions of the brain such as the hippocampus, neocortex and cerebellum.

Han et al. [30] used animal model APP/PSEN1, 30 female mice divided into 3 groups with 10 animals each: treatment group, positive control group, and negative control group. The therapeutic adopted was LED emitting infrared light for 6 minutes for a period of 40 days, and the animals were analyzed by the method of Morris Aquatic Labyrinth and the results by statistical analysis. The measured parameters were spatial memory and cognitive performance after treatment with LED. The results suggested that infrared therapy emitted by LED can improve the performance in spatial learning and memory capacity.

Han et al. [31] used animal model C57BL/6 J, being females divided into 3 groups: rats without irradiation (n = 10), rats with irradiation (n = 10), and normal rats without irradiation (n = 12). The therapeutic adopted was LED with wavelengths between 1040 nm and 1090 nm, power of 15 mW/cm2; 6 minutes a day, for 40 days, suspended for 28 days, and then starting the treatment again for another 15 days. The measured parameters were spatial memory and the presence of senile plaques after the LED treatment period. They found that LED is able of improving performance in spatial learning and moderately reduces senile plaques.

Eltchechem et al. [32] used 60 rats, 30 treated (GT group) and 30 in a control group (GC group). The treatment was with LED (627 nm 7 W/cm^2, 70 mV) in the frontal region, one time every day for 100 s for 21 days. The methods of analysis were Morris Aquatic Labyrinth, Open field, histological analysis, immuno-histochemical analysis, and statistical analysis. The measured parameters were the βA deposits in the GT in relation to the GC with 7, 14 and 21 days after LED irradiation. The results found were better movement, exploration, and spatial memory of the GT in relation to the CG.

Yue et al. [33] used APP/PS1 AD model mice treated, APP/PS1 control mice and healthy C57BL/6 mice as a negative control. The treatment was with photobiomodulation by LED 630 nm with application of 40 minutes and light intensity of 0.55 mW/cm2 in the skull and abdomen 5 days a week for 2 months. The methods of analysis were Morris Aquatic Labyrinth, fluorescent microscopy; magnetic resonance; biochemical analysis and statistical analysis. It was observed destruction of βA plaques group and activation of the formaldehyde dehydrogenase enzyme, that degrades formaldehyde, which acts by accelerating the deposition of βA in the extracellular space and, consequently, attenuation of βA aggregation facilitated by formaldehyde. In addition, the light reduced βA deposition in the extracellular space, positively influenced the flow of interstitial fluids and recovered cognitive functions in AD mice.

Cho et al. [34] evaluated the effect of photobiomodulation using 610 nm LED on amyloid plaques, gliosis, and neuronal loss to prevent and/or recover cognitive functions and the ideal time to start therapy. 5XFAD AD model rats were used, divided into a group that started therapy at 2 months old, and another at 6 months old. The treatment consisted of the simultaneous application of light in two places (midpoint of the parietal bone and midline of the seventh cervical vertebra) for 20 minutes, 3 times a week, for 14 weeks. From behavioral tests, immunohistochemical analysis and Western blot, it was found in the initial stages the reduction of the accumulation of amyloid plaques, neuronal loss and microgliosis, and the relief of cognitive dysfunction.

9.2.2 Resveratrol: Neuroprotective action

Yin et al. [35] investigated if resveratrol could mitigate the early loss induced by βA in the neuron excitability in the hippocampus and the mechanism involved on it. The excitability and the potassium currents dependent on the pyramidal neuron CA1 voltage of rats were analyzed using the whole-cell patch-clamp technique. The authors discovered that resveratrol reverted the increase of βA peptide and the increase induced in the frequency of the repetitive shots, mitigated the decrease induced by βA in the transitory potassium channels, and rectified the delay on neuron potassium channels. Besides, it was shown that resveratrol decreased the levels of kinase A (PKA) and inhibited the activation of the signaling path PI3K/Akt.

Sarroca et al. [36] assessed the beginning and progression of the pathology of Alzheimer's disease through a diet rich in fat (HFD) and the influence of resveratrol in this situation. Many evidences suggest that HFD increases the risk of Alzheimer's disease (AD), but the molecular mechanisms through which the HFD causes its negative effects on the brain and the pathophysiology of AD are still widely unknown. The authors used wild mice (WT) and AD 5XFAD transgenic (5XFAD mice represent an aggressive model of AD due to the exposure to intraneuronal β-amyloid-42 in 1,5 months, extracellular amyloid plaques in 2 months, gliosis in 2 months, memory deficits in 4 months and neuronal loss in 9 months) treated with a control diet of HFD (60% kcal of fat) or HFD supplemented with 0,1% of resveratrol for 16 weeks. From the analysis of behavioral tests, glucose intolerance tests, preparation of tissue samples, coloring with Thioflavin-S, Western Blotting, and proteasome activity test, it was possible to observe that the results showed the resveratrol reduced the amyloid load aggravated by HFD in 5XFAD model (model of Alzheimer's disease with a pathology of low tau protein), the analysis by Western Blotting showed thar the cortex tissue did not show modification in the levels of tau protein. However, HFD was responsible for inducing a significant increase in the levels of pTau in both WT and 5XFAD mice, and resveratrol indicated the ability to normalize the levels of pTau in both groups fed with HFD. Resveratrol also inhibited the amyloidogenic processing enhanced by HFD.

Ma et al. [37] reported that AD and diabetes mellitus (DM) usually coexist in patients because one increases the incidence of the other. In this context, the authors studied the neuroprotection induced by resveratrol in mice with DM and AD caused by the injection of streptozocin (intraperitoneal) and β-amyloid 1–40 (hippocampus). Through biochemical and immunological analysis it was demonstrated that resveratrol increased SIRT1 expression, inhibited memory damage, increased the levels of acetylcholinesterase (responsible for the hydrolysis of acetylcholine in cholinergic synapses), malondialdehyde (marker of oxidative stress), interleukin-1β and interleukin 6 (interleukin-1β acts in the hypothalamus stimulating the release of corticotrophin by the posterior pituitary gland and the corticotrophin acts on the anterior pituitary gland, releasing adrenocorticotrophic hormone, and interleukin 6 is responsible for the influence on the immunological responses, mediating the acute stage of the inflammation), and showed decreased levels of choline acetyltransferase (mediator of the synthesis of acetylcholine), superoxide dismutase (responsible for catalyzing the dismutation of the superoxide in oxygen and hydrogen peroxide, an important antioxidant defense), and glutathione (causes several antioxidants, neutralizes free radicals).

Corpas et al. [38] evaluated the neuroprotection effects of resveratrol in two groups of mice: non-transgenic control (NoTg) and AD transgenic model (3xTg-AD). Both groups were fed with a supplemented diet of 100 mg/kg from 2 months of age for 10 months. Using Western Blotting, behavior and cognitive tests and proteasome activity test, it was possible to analyze how resveratrol induced complete protection against memory loss and brain pathology in 3xTg-AD mice and induced a cognitive increase in healthy NoTg mice. It also reduced anxiety in both strains, reducing the presence of hippocampal βA and tau protein in 3xTg-AD. As for the proteostases analysis, an increase of the levels of the enzyme neprisilin was observed, being responsible for the degradation of β-amyloid, reduction of amyloidogenic secretase BACE1, increase of the levels of proteasome protein in both mice groups, vital role in the increasing of the adenosine kinase activated by monophosphate (AMPK) and the positive regulation of the SITR1 path.

Chen et al. [39] evaluated the levels of resveratrol in Tg6799 mice (transgenic model with five family mutations on Alzheimer's disease). The mice were divided in a group treated with resveratrol (solution 0.5%, 60 mg/kg) and a control group (treated with saline solution). The treatment was administered orally, daily, for 60 days. To interpret the results, the tests performed were the open field test, Y maze test, Morris aquatic labyrinth test, coloring with Thioflavin-S, ELISA Aβ40 and Aβ42 and finally Western Blotting, demonstrating that resveratrol reduced the disposition of the amyloid plaques, β-amyloid levels of −42 and β-secretase levels. Resveratrol also reduced the expression of the amyloid precursor protein and its cleavage products. Besides, there was a behavioral improvement related to the spatial working memory, according to the Y maze test, and improvement on the spatial memory deficits, evaluated by the Morris aquatic labyrinth test. However, resveratrol did not influence the motor function.

Wang et al. [40] used AD model rats (by hippocampal injection of β-amyloid 1–42) to investigate the possible effects of resveratrol on the behavior of spatial learning, memory and synaptic plasticity, as well as changes on the expression and phosphorylation of SIRT1 of the protein connecting to the response element of cyclic AMP (CREB). In addition to the already accepted analysis, protein extraction and Western Blotting were also done, and it was shown that resveratrol reverted the spatial learning memory damage evaluated by the Morris aquatic labyrinth, and to investigate the underlying mechanisms of the neuroprotector effects of resveratrol on the memory and learning, the long-term potentiation (LTP) was registered in the CA1 area of the hippocampus. So, it was demonstrated that the Aβ1–42 hippocampal injection did not affect significatively the basal excitatory post-synaptic potential (fEPSP), while Aβ1–42 suppressed the induction of hippocampal LTP. In addition to that, resveratrol avoided reductions on the expression of SIRT1 and phosphorylation of the cyclic AMP response element connecting protein (CREB).

10. Discussion

10.1 Transcranial photobiomodulation

LED is a radiation of varying wavelength, not coherent and which is standing out in the field of medical treatment and phototherapy for being an alternative to the high cost of laser therapy [41]. The use of light with Low-intensity Laser Therapy or by Light-emitting Diode is called photobiomodulation [42] and among its functions, it is the stimulation of neural activity, that occurs through interaction with cytochrome c oxidase (unit IV of the mitochondrial electrons transport chain), which through a series of reactions, stimulates the ATP synthase enzyme to produce more ATP, improving brain function [27]. LED, however, emerged as an innovation in the field because it does not give off heat, is portable, is easy to apply, and is more durable when compared to other methods such as laser therapy (**Figure 10**) [27].

Recent advances in optogenetics and the development of microscale LED platforms have elevated the viability of phototherapy for use on target brain cells [43]. The method in the treatment of neurodegenerative diseases is under development, and studies show that this therapy can act on amyloid aggregates [44, 45].

Although biological effects of the light emitted by the LED have been reported for a wide spectrum of wavelengths, the research related to the effects on the Alzheimer disease has focused on the wavelengths in the region of the nearby infrared. This approach involves the tissue irradiation with a low intensity light and promotes protective effects on the central nervous system [46].

In this approach, the primary photoreceptors are the mitochondria, and there is evidence that the action is responsible for preserving and restoring the function of the neurons by their action on the mitochondrial cytochrome *c* oxidase enzyme, which, due to a series of biochemical reactions, results in a greater production of ATP by the stimulation of the ATP synthase enzyme. Moreover, the effect is also related to the signaled pathways activated by reactive oxygen species, release of nitric oxide and increased cyclic adenosine monophosphate. Thus, these factors work together to produce effects in the regions in which the function was compromised by ischemia, traumatic injuries, and neurodegeneration [47].

Thus, both in animal models and in human patient trials, the treatment promotes satisfactory results. As for the studies described in the results and referring to those that used animal models, the photobiomodulation, with the different protocols tested, brought together some results. Results described in *in vivo* studies using animal models showed reduction of hyper phosphorylation of the tau protein, attenuation of neurofibrillary tangles, decreased oxidative stress markers, reduced deposition, number, and size of β-amyloid plaques, reduced neuronal loss, formaldehyde dehydrogenase activation, positive influence on the flow of interstitial fluids, and capacity to recover and improve cognitive functions, such as learning and spatial memory capacity [30–34].

Regarding the application places and treatment time in animal models, most of the studies focused on the transcranial application, except for the research by Yue et al. [33] who performed transcranial and abdominal application.

About treatment time, in general, irradiation protocols between 21 and 40 days were used, except in the study by Cho et al. [34] in which the treatment (both early and late) was carried out for 14 weeks, and represented a longer irradiation protocol, which differs from those established by other authors.

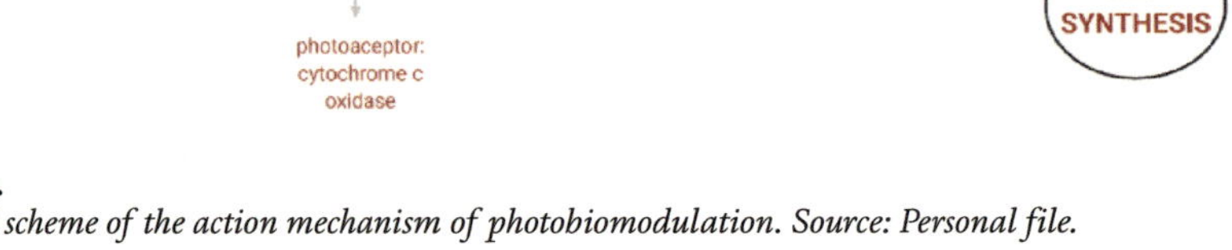

Figure 10.
Simplified scheme of the action mechanism of photobiomodulation. Source: Personal file.

In relation to human patients, the effects were mostly focused and described on mental and cognitive performance states. It was observed that the therapy provided a significant improvement in dementia, and presented cognitive functional increase, sleep improvement and fewer anxiety and anger outbreaks [27, 28]. It has also provided an increase in cerebral perfusion between the posterior cingulate cortex and the lateral parietal nodules in the network in a standard way [28].

The locations of application and time of treatment in clinical research were similar. Both studies that involved human models reported the use of transcranial and intranasal photobiomodulation. The treatment time did not differ either. A twelve-week protocol was adopted, which the only difference was in the post-treatment follow-up, with a period of four weeks without treatment being observed in the research by Saltmarche [27].

As for safety in the human model, the treatment was described as well tolerated and did not induce any adverse effects. These results support the therapeutic potential for viable treatment (including home treatment) of patients with dementias. However, larger, and more controlled studies are still necessary. It is indispensable, for consolidating the therapy, to clarify the ideal irradiation parameters such as application time, active treatment, and follow-up, as well as the general efficacy and safety profile [27, 28].

Regarding considerations for future research, they should be carried out by following longer and not discontinued treatment protocols. As according to Saltmarche [27] a period of four weeks without treatment, after initiation, resulted in deterioration of the positive effects achieved with twelve weeks of active treatment, and it caused difficulties for patients and caregivers. Furthermore, the author describes that the movement of patients to the clinic for LED applications caused stress. Therefore, for future work, home treatment is expected, which is possible considering the facility and viability of the application if it is properly oriented and performed.

Finally, it is interesting to use standardized cognitive assessments that consider different aspects, such as quality sleep, communication and social interaction, reduction of anxiety, depression, and disturbing behaviors to cover most of the effects induced by photobiomodulation.

10.2 Resveratrol

The importance of oxidative stress in AD has been increasingly recognized. Several studies have shown evidence that oxidative stress may contribute to the pathogenesis of AD through the formation of oxygen free radicals. Thus, the therapeutic focus has also been directed towards the use of antioxidants in the treatment of AD [10, 48].

Although antioxidants do not provide objective improvement in cognition, they can delay the natural evolution of the disease due to their supposed neuroprotective effect [48]. Polyphenols from food consumption plants have already been confirmed as neuroprotective compounds, including by a reduction on the aggregation of β-amyloid protein, such is the case of the trans-3,5,4′-trihydroxystylbene, Resveratrol [12].

Resveratrol is widely found in grapes used to produce red wine and in cereals and has been tested in different models of the disease (*in vitro* and *in vivo*), presenting neuroprotective effect and inhibiting the aggregation of βA [12].

Among its different proven forms of action, the following stand out: (a) competition with coenzyme Q to reduce the oxidative complex, the site of production of reactive oxygen species (ROS); (b) neutralization of oxygen free radicals formed; and (c) inhibition of lipid peroxidation induced by Fenton reaction products, in the mitochondria (**Figure 11**) [49].

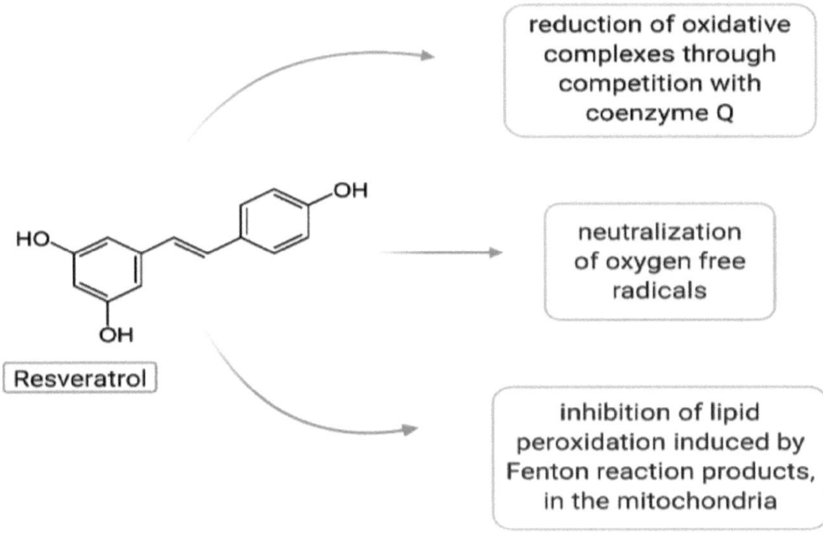

Figure 11.
Effects of resveratrol already proven. Source: Personal file.

In vitro studies have shown that Resveratrol has neuroprotective and preventive effects related to oxidative damage induced by β-amyloid and memory loss by reducing the accumulation of lipid peroxides, positive regulation of the endogenous antioxidants action and increased expression of memory associated proteins [50]. Although the effects of Resveratrol are mostly attributed to its antioxidant activity, studies suggest that its biological activity may be associated with different pathways. Yin et al. [35] demonstrated that Resveratrol act on the nervous system by inhibiting the electrical activity, relieving β-amyloid induced dysfunction in hippocampal CA1 pyramidal neurons, associating this effect with the ability to recover potassium currents.

In view of its ability to modulate potassium channels, Resveratrol plays a promising activity to attenuate neural impairments induced by β-amyloid. However, as the antioxidant has shown a variety of neuroprotective actions, it is also possible that other signals are involved, such as other ion channels, e.g., calcium and sodium channels, which can be exploited in the future to elucidate the effects achieved by Resveratrol due to the relationship with certain central nervous systems disorders [35].

Regarding the in vivo studies, the effects of resveratrol were already expressed and described in different ways, and among them the ones of note are reduction of amyloid load and inhibition of the amyloidogenic processing [37–39], neuroprotection of memory loss, cognitive improvement and acetylcholinesterase inhibition [38, 39], anxiety reduction, increase on the AMPK levels [36, 39], positive regulation of the SIRT1 path [37–40] and reversion of the damage on spatial memory [39, 41].

As a future perspective, based on the neuroprotectant activities observed in vitro and in vivo, it is expected that clinical trials are done with long term treatments and low formulations with improved pharmacokinetic properties (due to the low availability shown) to sustain the possibility of a therapeutic alternative for the treatment of AD, as well as the clarification of its mechanisms of action, safety and efficiency.

11. Conclusion

Thus, it is concluded that both the treatment with Transcranial Photobiomodulation using LEDs as light sources, and the treatment with

Resveratrol have numerous benefits that can be useful in the treatment of AD. However, there is a need for new research that covers interventions with greater specificity and control, so that the ideal doses and treatment protocols are defined.

Author details

Ivo Ilvan Kerppers[1]*, Andressa Panegalli Hosni[2], Andressa Leticia Miri[3], Maria Elvira Ribeiro Cordeiro[1], Flávio Klinpovous Kerppers[1], Mariane Maria Silveira Vieira de Lima[4], Ana Carolina Dorigoni Bini[2], Felipe Figueiredo Moreira[1], Patricia Pacheco Tyski Suckow[2], Eliane Gonçalves de Jesus Fonseca[2], Larissa Sakis Bernardi[1] and Paulo Renato de Oliveira[1]

1 State University of the Center-West, Guarapuava, PR, Brazil

2 Postgraduate Program in Pharmaceutical Sciences, State University of the Center-West, Guarapuava, PR, Brazil

3 Postgraduate Program in Rehabilitation Science, State University of Londrina, Londrina, PR, Brazil

4 Postgraduate Program in Nanoscience and Bioscience, State University of the Center-West, Guarapuava, PR, Brazil

*Address all correspondence to: ikerppers@hotmail.com

References

[1] Tarawneh R, Holtzman DM. O problema clínico da doença de Alzheimer sintomática e comprometimento cognitivo leve. Cold Spring Harb Perspect Med. 2012; 2 (5): a006148.

[2] Alzheimer's Disease International. London, SE1 0BB, UK.

[3] Arora K, Alfulaij N, Higa JK, Panee J, Nichols RA. Impact of Sustained Exposure to β-Amyloid on Calcium Homeostasis and Neuronal Integrity in Model Nerve Cell System Expressing α4β2 Nicotinic Acetylcholine Receptors. Journal of Biological Chemistry. 2013; (16):11175-11190.

[4] Daulatzai MA. Fundamental role of pan-inflammation and oxidative-nitrosative pathways in neuropathogenesis of Alzheimer's disease. Am. J. Neurodegener. 2016; (5): 1-28.

[5] Kumar A, Sharma V, Singh VP, Kaundal M, Gupta MK, Bariwal J, et al. Herbs to curb cyclic nucleotide phosphodiesterase and their potential role in Alzheimer's disease. Mechanisms of Ageing and Development. 2015; (149):75-87.

[6] C. Vickers J, Mitew S, Woodhouse A, M. Fernandez-Martos C, T. Kirkcaldie M, J. Canty A, et al. Defining the earliest pathological changes of Alzheimer's disease. CAR. 2016; (3):281-7.

[7] McKhann GM, Knopman DS, Chertkow H, Hyman BT, Jack CR, Kawas CH, et al. The diagnosis of dementia due to Alzheimer's disease: Recommendations from the National Institute on Aging-Alzheimer's Association workgroups on diagnostic guidelines for Alzheimer's disease. Alzheimer's & Dementia. 2011;(3):263-269.

[8] Apostolova LG. Alzheimer Disease: CONTINUUM: Lifelong Learning in Neurology. 2016; (2, Dementia):419-34.

[9] Pearson HA, Peers C. Physiological roles for amyloid β peptides: Physiological roles for amyloid β peptides. The Journal of Physiology. 2006;575(1):5-10.

[10] Baptista JDS. New therapeutic approaches for Alzheimer's disease (Doctoral dissertation). 2019.

[11] Falco AD, Cukierman DS, Hauser-Davis RA, Rey NA. Alzheimer's disease: etiological hypotheses and prospects for treatment. New Chemistry. 2016. (1):63-80.

[12] Fridman C, Gregório SP, Dias Neto E, Ojopi ÉPB. Genetic changes in Alzheimer's disease. Archives of Clinical Psychiatry. 2004; (1): 19-25.

[13] Paula VJR de, Guimarães FM, Forlenza OV. Papel da proteína Tau na fisiopatologia da demência frontotemporal. Rev psiquiatr clín. 2009;36(5):197-202.

[14] Dalmagro AP, Cazarin CA, Zenaide F dos S. Atualização no estudo das bases bioquímicas e moleculares da doença de Alzheimer. BASR. 2020;(1):118-130.

[15] Blennow K, de Leon MJ, Zetterberg H. Alzheimer's disease. The Lancet. julho de 2006; (9533):387-403.

[16] Bush AI. Drug Development Based on the Metals Hypothesis of Alzheimer's Disease. Chohan MO, organizador. JAD. 2008; (2):223-40.

[17] Bush AI, Tanzi RE. Therapeutics for Alzheimer's disease based on the metal hypothesis. Neurotherapeutics. 2008; (3):421-432.

[18] Urbanc B, Betnel M, Cruz L, Li H, Fradinger EA, Monien BH, et al.

Structural Basis for Aβ1-42 Toxicity Inhibition by Aβ C-Terminal Fragments: Discrete Molecular Dynamics Study. Journal of Molecular Biology. 2011; (2):316-328.

[19] Danysz W, Parsons CG. Alzheimer's disease, β-amyloid, glutamate, NMDA receptors and memantine - searching for the connections: Alzheimer's disease, β-amyloid, glutamate, NMDA receptors and memantine. British Journal of Pharmacology. 2012; (2):324-352.

[20] Schnabel J. Amyloid: Little proteins, big clues. Nature. 2011; (7355):S12-4. BRESSAN RA, PILOWSKY LS. Hipótese glutamatérgica da esquizofrenia. Brazilian Journal of Psychiatry, v. 25, n. 3, p. 177-183, 2003.

[21] Kása P, Rakonczay Z, Gulya K. The cholinergic system in Alzheimer's disease. Prog Neurobiol. 1997; (6):511-535.

[22] Green A, Ellis K, Ellis J, Bartholomeusz C, Ilic S, Croft R, et al. Muscarinic and nicotinic receptor modulation of object and spatial - back working memory in humans. Pharmacology Biochemistry and Behavior. 2005; (3):575-584.

[23] Ferreira ST, Clarke JR, Bomfim TR, De Felice FG. Inflammation, defective insulin signaling, and neuronal dysfunction in Alzheimer's disease. Alzheimers Dement. 2014; (1 Suppl):S76-83.

[24] Craft S, Watson GS. Insulin and neurodegenerative disease: shared and specific mechanisms. Lancet Neurol. 2004; (3):169-178.

[25] Bomfim TR, Forny-Germano L, Sathler LB, Brito-Moreira J, Houzel JC, Decker H, Silverman MA, Kazi H, Melo HM, McClean PL, Holscher C, ArnoldSE,TalbotK,KleinWL,MunozDP, Ferreira ST, De Felice FG. An anti-diabetes agent protects the mouse brain from defective insulin signaling caused by Alzheimer's disease- associated Aβ oligomers. J Clin Invest. 2012; (4):1339-1353.

[26] Talbot K, Wang HY, Kazi H, Han LY, Bakshi KP, Stucky A, Fuino RL, Kawaguchi KR, Samoyedny AJ, Wilson RS, Arvanitakis Z, Schneider JA, Wolf BA, Bennett DA, Trojanowski JQ, Arnold SE. Demonstrated brain insulin resistance in Alzheimer's disease patients is associated with IGF-1 resistance, IRS-1 dysregulation, and cognitive decline. J Clin Invest. 2012; (4):1316-1338.

[27] Saltmarche AE, Naeser MA, Ho KF, Hamblin MR, Lim L. Significant Improvement in Cognition in Mild to Moderately Severe Dementia Cases Treated with Transcranial Plus Intranasal Photobiomodulation: Case Series Report. Photomedicine and Laser Surgery. 2017 Aug;35(8):432-441.

[28] Chao LL. Effects of home photobiomodulation treatments on cognitive and behavioral function, cerebral perfusion and resting functional connectivity in patients with dementia: a pilot study. Photobiomodulation, Photomedicine, Laser Surg. 2019. 37, 133-141.

[29] Purushothuman S, Johnstone DM, Nandasena C, van Eersel J, Ittner LM, Mitrofanis J, et al. Near infrared light mitigates cerebellar pathology in transgenic mouse models of dementia. Neuroscience Letters. 2015. (591):155-159.

[30] Han M, Wang Q, Zeng Y, Meng Q, Zhang J, Wei X. Studying infra-red-light therapy for treating Alzheimer' s disease. 2016. SPIE 9709, 1-6.

[31] Han M, Wang Q, Wang X, Zeng Y, Huang Y, Meng Q, et al. Near infra-red-light treatment of Alzheimer's disease. J Innov Opt Health Sci. 2018; (01):1750012.

[32] Eltchechem CL, Salgado ASI, Zângaro RA, da Silva Pereira MC, Kerppers II, da Silva LA, et al. Transcranial LED therapy on amyloid-β toxin 25-35 in the hippocampal region of rats. Lasers Med Sci. 2017; (4):749-756.

[33] Yue X, Mei Y, Zhang Y, Tong Z, Cui D, Yang J, Wang A, Wang R, Fei X, Ai L, Di Y, Luo H, Li H, Luo W, Lu Y, Li R, Duan C, Gao G, Tong Z. New insight into Alzheimer's disease: light reverses the flow of interstitial fluid obstructed by Aβ and improves memory decline in APP/PS1 mice. Alzheimer's Dement. Transl. Res. Clin. Interv. 2019; (5): 671-684.

[34] Cho GM, Lee S-Y, Park JH, Kim MJ, Park K-J, Choi BT, Shim Y-I, Kim NG, Shin HK. Photobiomodulation using a low-level LED improves cognitive dysfunction in the 5XFAD mouse model of Alzheimer's disease. J Gerontol A Biol Sci Med Sci. 2020; (75):631-639.

[35] Yin H, Wang H, Zhang H, Gao N, Zhang T, Yang Z. Resveratrol Attenuates Aβ-Induced Early Hippocampal Neuron Excitability Impairment via Recovery of Function of Potassium Channels. Neurotox Res. outubro de 2017; (3):311-324.

[36] Sarroca S, Gatius A, Rodríguez-Farré E, Vilchez D, Pallàs M, Griñán-Ferré C, et al. Resveratrol confers neuroprotection against high-fat diet in a mouse model of Alzheimer's disease via modulation of proteolytic mechanisms. The Journal of Nutritional Biochemistry. 2021; (89):108569.

[37] Ma X, Sun Z, Han X, Li S, Jiang X, Chen S, et al. Neuroprotective Effect of Resveratrol via Activation of Sirt1 Signaling in a Rat Model of Combined Diabetes and Alzheimer's Disease. Front Neurosci. 2020; (13):1400.

[38] Copas R, Griñán-Ferré C, Rodríguez-Farré E, Pallàs M, Sanfeliu C. Resveratrol Induces Brain Resilience Against Alzheimer Neurodegeneration Through Proteostasis Enhancement. Mol Neurobiol. 2019; (2):1502-1516.

[39] Chen Y, Shi GW, Liang ZM, Sheng SY, Shi YS, Peng L, Wang YP, Wang F, Zhang XM. Resveratrol improves cognition and decreases amyloid plaque formation in Tg6799 mice. Mol Med Rep. 2019; (5):3783-3790.

[40] Wang R, Zhang Y, Li J, Zhang C. Resveratrol ameliorates spatial learning memory impairment induced by Aβ1-42 in rats. Neuroscience. 2017; (344):39-47.

[41] Santos KMMG, Cordeiro MER, da Silva Pereira MC, Barbosa D, Pezzini AA, Kerppers II. Comparative study in photodynamic therapy using the same photosensitizer in tissue repair after second-degree burns in an experimental model. Laser Dent Sci. 2020; (1):17-24.

[42] Kerppers FK, Dos Santos KMMG, Cordeiro MER, da Silva Pereira MC, Barbosa D, Pezzini AA, Cunha LF, Fonseca M, Bragnholo K, Salgado ASI, Kerppers II. Study of transcranial photobiomodulation at 945-nm wavelength: anxiety and depression. Lasers Med Sci. 2020; (9):1945-1954.

[43] Kim T -i., McCall JG, Jung YH, Huang X, Siuda ER, Li Y, et al. Injectable, Cellular-Scale Optoelectronics with Applications for Wireless Optogenetics. Science. 2013; (6129):211-216.

[44] Liao Y-H, Chang Y-J, Yoshiike Y, Chang Y-C, Chen Y-R. Negatively Charged Gold Nanoparticles Inhibit Alzheimer's Amyloid-β Fibrillization, Induce Fibril Dissociation, and Mitigate Neurotoxicity. Small. 2012; (23):3631-3639.

[45] Taniguchi A, Shimizu Y, Oisaki K, Sohma Y, Kanai M. Switchable photooxygenation catalysts that sense

higher-order amyloid structures. Nature Chem. 2016; (10):974-982.

[46] Purushothuman S, Johnstone DM, Nandasena C, Mitrofanis J, Stone J. Photobiomodulation with near infrared light mitigates Alzheimer's disease-related pathology in cerebral cortex – evidence from two transgenic mouse models. Alzheimers. Res. 2014; (6): 1-13.

[47] Naeser MA, Hamblin MR. Potential for Transcranial Laser or LED Therapy to Treat Stroke, Traumatic Brain Injury, and Neurodegenerative Disease. Photomedicine and Laser Surgery. 2011; (7):443-446.

[48] Barros PP, Gonçalves GMS, Silva GHD, Bastos MCVD, Ramos LN, Fernandes MM. Lycopene and resveratrol pretreatment did not interfere with the liver of hepatectomized rats. Acta Cirurgica Brasileira. 2017; (3):194-202.

[49] Rege S, Geetha T, L Broderick T, Ramesh Babu J. Resveratrol protects β amyloid-induced oxidative damage and memory associated proteins in H19-7 hippocampal neuronal cells. Current Alzheimer Research. 2015; (2):147-156.

[50] Sousa JC e, Santana ACF, Magalhães GJP. Resveratrol in Alzheimer's disease: a review of pathophysiology and therapeutic potential. Arq Neuro-Psiquiatr. 2020; (8):501-511.

Chapter 4

Diagnosis of Cardiac Amyloidosis Using Non-Invasive Technics

Eva Strickler, Ernest Tsiaze, Gerrit Hellige, Dominik Zumstein, Dominik Waldmeier and Nisha Arenja

Abstract

Amyloidosis is a rare multiorgan disease defined by a process of irreversible, extracellular accumulation of fibrillar proteins in the tissues, including the heart. Cardiac involvement is seen in most forms of amyloidosis, but it is frequently present and clinically significant in light chain (AL)-amyloidosis as well as transthyretin amyloidosis (ATTR). Cardiac amyloid accumulation leads to a restrictive filling pattern, which must be differentiated from other forms of restrictive and hypertrophic cardiomyopathies due to consequences for the treatment. Evolving knowledge of the disease has led to a definite diagnosis of the cardiac amyloidosis (CA) using non-invasive and low-risk diagnostic features, such as scintigraphy (gamma scan) and cardiovascular magnetic resonance (CMR) imaging using late gadolinium enhancement (LGE) and T1 mapping technics. The availability and diagnostic accuracy of these technics has reduced the need for cardiac biopsy. In the following chapter, we will describe common types of CA, the basic concepts, and updates of non-invasive diagnostic features.

Keywords: Cardiac Amyloidosis, Diagnosis, Non-Invasive Technics, Imaging Modalities

1. Introduction

1.1 Common types of amyloidosis

Amyloidosis is an infiltrative disease defined by extracellular accumulation of fibrillar proteins in the tissues, including the heart (cardiac amyloidosis (CA)). Lately, about 30 different types of amyloidosis have been described, each due to a specific misfolded protein [1]. Some types of amyloidosis are hereditary others are caused by abnormal organ or plasma cells producing a precursor protein. Additional causes involve long-term dialysis or inflammatory diseases. The disease is classified as "localized amyloidosis" and "systemic amyloidosis".

The main subtypes of amyloidosis are summarized in the following:

- **Light chain amyloidosis (AL, primary amyloidosis)**: AL-amyloidosis represents the most common type of amyloidosis with a prevalence of >0.3 per 100,000 of the general population. The incidence is estimated at 8.9–12.7 per million person-years [2]. The age at manifestation is usually between 60 and 69 years. Precursor protein in AL-amyloidosis is a misfolded immunoglobulin light chain produced by plasma cells. Deposition of misfolded proteins can

 IntechOpen

occur in virtually any organ system. However, in most cases, the heart and kidneys are involved. Cardiac involvement is described in more than 70% of the cases with a mortality rate of up to 50% per year after the first episode of an acute heart failure [3]. The development of AL cardiomyopathy is caused by the AL amyloid-associated lysosomal dysfunction, oxidative stress, and induction of autophagy (direct toxicity) [4].

- **Amyloid transthyretin (ATTR)-amyloidosis**: ATTR-amyloidosis is a life-threatening and progressive type of amyloidosis. Two forms of ATTR can be distinguished, the mutant transthyretin (**ATTRm**, referred to as familial or hereditary transthyretin amyloidosis (FTA)) and the wild-type amyloidosis (**ATTRwt**, known as well as senile systemic amyloidosis). The precursor protein is amyloid transthyretin (TTR), a transport protein, which usually carries thyroid hormone thyroxine (T4) and retinol-binding protein bound to retinol in serum and cerebrospinal fluid.

- **ATTRm** is an autosomal dominant condition caused by mutations in the TTR gene with abnormal secreted by the liver and deposited in various organs. The type and severity of organ involvement defines its prognosis. ATTRm is clinically heterogeneous and causes a broad spectrum of symptoms. Most often patients suffer from mixed clinical phenotype consisting of sensory and motor impairment and multiple organ failure [5]. Although the exact prevalence of ATTRm is unknown, recently published data reported a global prevalence as high as 38,000 persons [5]. In African Americans ATTR-CA is frequently associated with the mutation Val142Ile (formerly known as Val122Ile), which is carried by 10% of African Americans with heart failure with reduced ejection fraction (HFrEF) and by 1.5–3.5% of the general African American population [6]. In the general Caucasian population this mutation is extremely rare (< 0.005%) [7, 8].

- **ATTRwt** is the most common cause of CA, particularly in the elderly. In a population-based autopsy study Tanskanen M, et al. showed its presence in 25% of subjects aged >85 years [9]. Several studies presented concomitant ATTRwt-amyloidosis in patients with severe aortic stenosis and heart failure with preserved ejection fraction (HFpEF) [10]. The prevalence among patients, who underwent transcatheter aortic valve implantation (TAVI) was reported in 8–16% [11]. However, the prevalence in patients with (paradoxical) low-flow, low-gradient aortic stenosis was reported much higher, with up to 30% [12]. The amyloid protein is being stored in every structure of the heart including myocardium, valves, and coronary arteries. The accumulation of dysfunctional proteins in the extracellular space of the myocardium leads to stiffening of the muscle and impairs the diastolic function of the heart. Heart failure occurs due to a restrictive filling pattern and impaired systolic function. Common arrhythmias resulting from structural changes usually include atrial fibrillation, atrioventricular block (AV), and sudden cardiac death (SCD) due to bradyarrhythmia or tachyarrhythmia [13].

- **Serum amyloid A amyloidosis (SAA, secondary amyloidosis)**: An acute-phase protein produced in the liver represents the precursor protein of SAA. An inflammatory disease, such as autoimmune and autoinflammatory disease, chronic infections, or cancer disease may trigger its production. The most commonly affected organs are the kidneys, liver and spleen. Cardiac involvement in SAA is rarely described in the literature [14].

- **Localized amyloidosis**: In localized amyloidosis the amyloidogenic protein is deposited at the site of production and not transported via bloodstream. Localized amyloidosis is usually light chain associated, but also serum amyloid A protein and TTR have been reported as localized disease. Localized immunoglobulin AL-amyloidosis is a rare disease. In a large study by the Mayo clinic 403 of 5551 AL patients (7%) were found for localized immunoglobulin AL-amyloidosis [15]. In this study, the median follow-up for survival and progression were 72 and 39 months. Localized amyloidosis is characterized by deposition of amyloid in a limited area of an anatomical region, such as isolated atrial amyloidosis caused by the precursor protein of atrial natriuretic factor (ANF) [16]. All tissues may be involved, but localized amyloidosis typically involves the laryngo-tracheobronchial tree, skin and urogenital tract.

1.2 Cardiac amyloidosis

CA is a leading cause of restrictive cardiomyopathy due to interstitial deposits of amyloid impairing the elasticity and contractility of the myocardium and leaving

Amyloid subtype	Precursor protein	Origin	Affected Organs	Clinical signs	Therapy
Light chain amyloidosis (AL)	Mono-clonal light chain	Plasma cells in bone marrow	Heart, kidneys, liver, nerves, gastro-intestinal tract, liver, soft tissue	periorbital hematoma, macro-glossia, proteinuria, weight loss	Chemotherapy
Hereditary transthyretin variant amyloidosis (ATTRm, familial or hereditary transthyretin amyloidosis (FTA))	Trans-thyretin mutation	Liver	Heart, kidneys, peripheral and autonomic nervous system, gastro-intestinal tract	Sudden cardiac death, arrhythmia, syncope, dysautonomia (orthostatic hypotension) peripheral sensory-motor neuropathy	Tafamidis, or 2-(3,5-dichloro-phenyl)-benzoxazole 6-carboxylic acid; Promising pharmacologic strategies to stabilize TTR
Transthyretin wild-type amyloidosis (ATTRwt, senile systemic amyloidosis)	Abnormal Trans-thyretin	Liver	Heart and peripheral nervous system	Heart failure, spinal stenosis, bilateral carpal tunnel syndrome	
Amyloid A amyloidosis	Serum amyloid A	Liver	Liver, kidneys, heart (rare)	Heart failure	Treatment of underlying inflammatory process
Apolipo-protein AA amyloidosis	Mutation in Apolipo-protein A1 gene		Liver, kidneys, heart	Heart failure, proteinuria, hematuria, edema, hepato-splenomegaly	Liver transplantation
Isolated atrial amyloidosis	Atrial natriuretic factor	Heart	Heart only	atrial fibrillation/ arrhythmia	no specific therapy available

Table 1.
Overview of the main subtypes of amyloidosis with the possibility of cardiac involvement.

the muscle stiff. Early findings include abnormal myocardial relaxation, gradually advancing to restrictive filling pattern, with signs and symptoms of heart failure. As specified above, the most common types of CA are AL and ATTR-amyloidosis (**Table 1**). An early diagnosis is of paramount importance in order to start the adequate treatment according to the disease, which determines the patient's prognosis.

Previously, the gold standard of CA diagnosis was a histological analysis of endomyocardial tissue. The invasive nature of an endomyocardial biopsy (EMB) limits its routine application. The following immediate or late complications are associated with EMB: pericardial effusion with or without tamponade, arrhythmias, tricuspid valve damage, pneumothorax, pulmonary embolism, nerve paralysis, bleeding complications, creation of an arteriovenous fistula, venous thromboembolism, and infections [17]. Major complications caused by EMB are described with a rate of 1% even when performed in large centers by experienced operators [18–20]. The cause of death is often perforation with tamponade.

Advances in imaging protocols have led to them being primarily used in daily clinical routine. The following chapter provides diagnostic steps for patients with CA including the most recent literature.

2. Non-invasive diagnostic techniques

2.1 Standard 12-lead electrocardiography (ECG) and Holter-ECG monitoring

The diagnostic procedure starts with a simple electrocardiogram (ECG), which may already provide clues for the presence of CA. Historically, CA is a condition associated with low voltage in the ECG, which usually is defined as a peak-to-peak QRS amplitude of less than 5 millimeters in the limb leads and/or less than 10 millimeters in the precordial leads [21].

Rapezzi et al. analyzed ECG recordings of AL, ATTRm and ATTRwt-amyloidosis and found significant differences among the three groups for low QRS voltage and left bundle-branch block [22]. Left bundle-branch block was frequently present in ATTRwt (40%), while in AL low QRS voltage was more common (25% ATTR versus 60% in AL). Boldrini et al. assessed the prevalence of intraventricular and atrioventricular conduction delays in a cohort of 344 AL patients. Intraventricular conduction delay due to myocardial amyloid deposits was associated with worse systolic function, higher mortality, and higher levels of cardiac biomarker [23]. Further 276 patients with a diagnosis of systemic amyloidosis, admitted to the Beijing Union Medical College Hospital from January 2000 to December 2011, were evaluated by Cheng and colleagues [24]. The study reported atrial arrhythmia, low voltage on limb leads, AV-block, and pseudo-infarct pattern as the most present ECG pattern in CA than control groups. In summary, the study data suggests a high specificity and a positive predictive value of low voltage on limb leads and pseudo-infarct pattern for the diagnosis of CA. However, these features are only observed in some CA patients (50% AL and 30% ATTR) and often in a later stage of the disease [25].

The most frequent arrhythmias in CA are atrial fibrillation (45–65%), ventricular tachyarrhythmias (ventricular tachycardia 9.9% and ventricular fibrillation 0.7%) and AV conduction delays (3.5%) [26]. The risk of SCD is increased, especially in advanced disease. The Austrian hot spot mutation His108Arg is linked to an increased incidence of ventricular tachycardia [27]. The proarrhythmic substrate for ventricular arrhythmias in CA is left ventricular fibrosis leading to micro- and macro-reentrant circuits [28]. Therefore, Holter-ECG monitoring is recommended in CA at initial presentation and follow-up.

Although electrophysiological studies (EPS) do not serve as a diagnostic tool, research supports their prognostic relevance. For example, in a study by Reisinger et al., 92% had a prolonged His-ventricular (HV) interval (>55 ms), which was identified as an independent predictor of SCD on multivariate analysis among patients with AL [29]. In a recently published study by Orini et al., ventricular conduction and repolarization abnormalities were more pronounced in AL compared to ATTR-amyloidosis [30].

In conclusion, in patients with AL and ATTR-amyloidosis, ECG and Holter-monitor are important tools to diagnose AV conduction delays as well as atrial and ventricular arrhythmias. Implantation of a permanent pacemaker system is recommended in patients meeting the established criteria for device implantation [31]. EPS should be considered in the setting of unexplained syncope due to the fact of common HV prolongation in absence of AV-Block in the 12-lead ECG. Patients with AL-amyloidosis have a higher risk to develop arrhythmias and suffer from a poor prognosis. However, implantable cardioverter defibrillator (ICD) for primary prophylactic therapy did not show a survival benefit in AL-CA. Their use may be considered in patients with AL or ATTR associated CA complicated with ventricular arrhythmias causing hemodynamic instability, who are having a life expectancy of more than one year with good functional status [32–34].

2.2 Cardiac biomarker and laboratory parameter

In suspected CA further laboratory parameters are needed. Due to an underlying plasma cell dyscrasia in AL-amyloidosis, a monoclonal gammopathy is detected by electrophoresis and immunochemical measurements of specific isotypes or free light chains (FLC) pairs. The spike of light chains is referred as "Bence Jones protein". For detection of even small amounts of FLC a serum fluorescence lifetime correlation spectroscopy and a serum FLC (sFLC) assay are of great additional value [35]. If monoclonal proteins are identified, the patient should be referred to a hematologist for further evaluation including a bone marrow biopsy. In case, an AL-amyloidosis can be ruled out, the next step should involve Technetium (Tc) -labeled cardiac scintigraphy (for further details see chapter 2.5).

Incorporation of sFLC differentiation into the current staging system for AL-amyloidosis improves risk stratification therapy optimization. Increased values of cardiac biomarkers such as brain natriuretic peptide (BNP), N-terminal brain natriuretic peptide (NT-proBNP), and Troponin (TnI, TnT) are used as screening parameters for cardiac involvement and clinical outcome. They might also assess the treatment response. In general, natriuretic peptides and Troponin levels are commonly elevated in CA, with a mild elevation seen in ATTR and higher levels in AL due to a cardiotoxic effect of light chains. The Mayo classification consists of TnT, NT-proBNP, and FLC-ratio (difference between light chain kappa and lambda) and helps estimating cardiac involvement and prognosis in AL patients [36].

2.3 Echocardiography

Echocardiography is an essential screening tool for CA and speeds up diagnosis. The most important finding represents the ventricular hypertrophy associated with amyloid self-aggregation (**Figure 1**). However, left ventricular (LV) wall thickening may also be seen in other conditions, such as long-standing arterial hypertension, high-grade aortic stenosis, hypertrophic cardiomyopathy (HCM) or storage diseases such as Fabry's disease. Therefore, further echocardiographic characteristics such as thickening of the atrial septum, valvular leaflets, as well as enlarged atria and pericardial effusion raise suspicion towards CA. Furthermore, assessment of

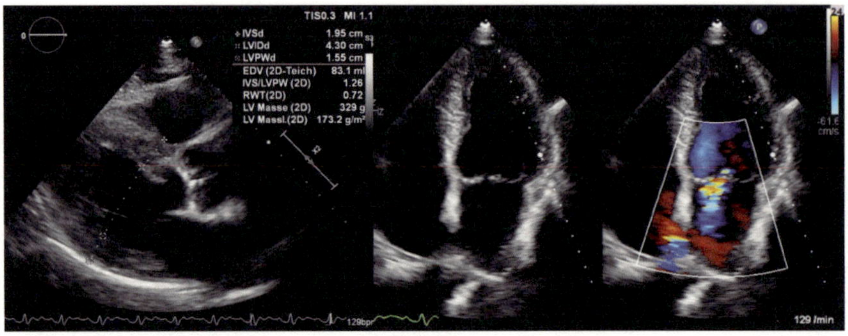

Figure 1.
Echocardiographic imaging showing a parasternal long axis view of a left ventricular hypertrophy and an apical 4-chamber view demonstrating mitral regurgitation.

diastolic function is a useful evaluation tool for CA. Diastolic dysfunction usually appears before pathologic measurements of left or right ventricular (RV) walls and it is the hallmark of amyloid heart disease [37]. A restrictive filling pattern is found in up to one-third of the CA population. According to the European classification of cardiomyopathies, CA may be regarded either as restrictive or hypertrophic cardiomyopathy based on the severity of diastolic filling impairment [38]. Based on hypertrophy and diastolic function parameters Aimo et al. developed a simple score named AMYLoidosis Index (AMYLI), as the product of relative wall thickness (RWT) and E/e' ratio, for initial screening of CA patients (AMYLI <2.22 excludes the diagnosis in patients undergoing a diagnostic screening for CA) [39]. However, this score needs further validation and is currently not in use for clinical routine.

Historically, "sparkling myocardium" is associated with CA. Granular sparkling is seen in approximately 25% of CA patients, which is attributed to increased echogenicity of the amyloid protein [40]. However, scanning with tissue harmonic frequencies imparts increased echogenicity of myocardium in general and granular sparkling may be overdiagnosed. In general, "speckled appearance" alone is not diagnostic of CA, since HCM, end-stage renal disease, harmonic imaging, and glycogen storage disease produce similar appearance [41].

Speckle tracking as an advanced echocardiography technic is a useful tool to differentiate CA from other causes of LV hypertrophy including other storage diseases. Myocardial speckle tracking-based strain imaging of the LV can help in the differential diagnosis and the presence of relative apical sparing may indicate CA. While left ventricular ejection fraction (LVEF) is preserved at early stages of CA, the longitudinal systolic contraction is already impaired [40]. Typically, the longitudinal strain at the basal and the mid ventricular segments is reduced, while the longitudinal apical strain of the LV is preserved (apical sparing). Preserved apical strain can be visualized using the strain ratio or the bull's eye plot (**Figure 2**) [42]. The pathophysiological basis of the apical sparing is not fully understood, but advanced imaging has shown evidence of amyloid deposition preferably in the basal and mid ventricular segments. In addition, a normal value of the global longitudinal strain (GLS) is known as a positive predictor for survival [43].

Although concomitant RV free wall hypertrophy is suggestive of infiltrative cardiomyopathy, an additional RV apical sparing pattern has been shown to distinguish CA from other storage diseases. Arvidsson et al. examined RV global and segmental strain of 42 subjects with ATTR amyloidosis. Patients with ATTR amyloidosis showed an apex-to-base RV strain gradient with relative apical sparing [44], RV involvement has been shown to occur most commonly after LV infiltration and has implications for prognosis [45].

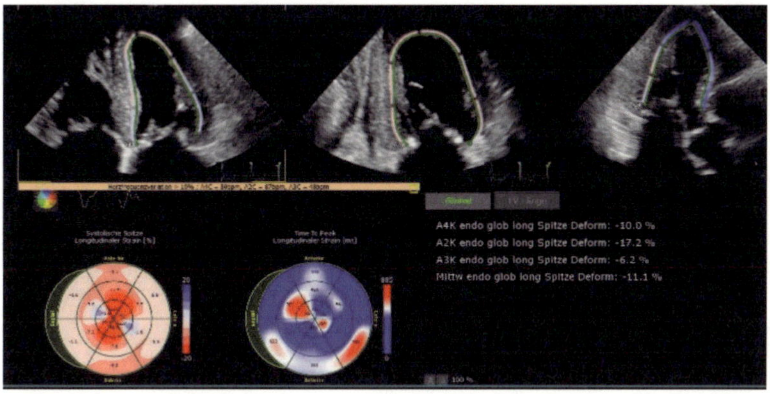

Figure 2.
Automated strain imaging using speckle-tracking algorithm.

To distinguish CA from other storage diseases, the following echocardiographic features may be helpful: presence of LV thickening, enlargement of the left atrium with wall thickening, lower E/e′, longer transmitral early filling wave deceleration time, reduced longitudinal strain in all myocardial segments with presence of relative apical sparing, additional RV hypertrophy with apical sparing pattern and mild pericardial and pleural effusion.

In summary, echocardiography using standard and speckle tracking imaging can provide many features suggesting amyloid heart disease though none of them are absolutely specific and further diagnostic tests are needed to accurately diagnose CA. Nevertheless, the presence of several echocardiographic findings increases the likelihood of the diagnosis, especially the combination of increased wall-thickness of the non-dilated LV with a restrictive filling pattern, biatrial enlargement, thickened valves, and pericardial effusion.

2.4 Cardiovascular magnetic resonance (CMR)

If echocardiographic findings hint at the presence of CA, cardiovascular magnetic resonance (CMR) is used to provide further support for the suspected diagnosis by evaluation of cardiac function and morphology using steady-state free precession (SSFP) sequences, tissue characterization via late gadolinium enhancement (LGE) and T1 mapping. CMR can characterize amyloid deposition in the extracellular tissue via LGE. In general, the phenomenon of LGE is explained by higher regional gadolinium concentration in the extracellular space and reduced distribution kinetics than in normal myocardium. In CA, the interstitium is substantially expanded by amyloid fiber accumulation, which is demonstrated by LGE in the myocardium with a dominant subendocardial distribution (**Figure 3**) [46, 47]. In a study by Pennell et al., a diffuse subendocardial LGE was observed in 69% [48]. Next to subendocardial different, other distribution patterns, ranging from the global transmural LGE to patchy focal LGE, have been described. The differences in the LGE pattern, especially the "patchy distribution" was explained by incorrect TI settings [49].

Suboptimal "myocardial nulling" is characteristic of CA. It describes the impossibility of adjustment of inversion time to discriminate the blood pool from the myocardium. An inversion recovery pulse sequence is used to null the myocardial signal during delayed-enhanced imaging. Usually, the blood pool reaches the null point before normal myocardium. However, this relationship is reversed in CA. Phase-sensitive inversion recovery (PSIR) reconstruction is emerging as the most accurate method to overcome this problem and assess LGE in CA. This technique

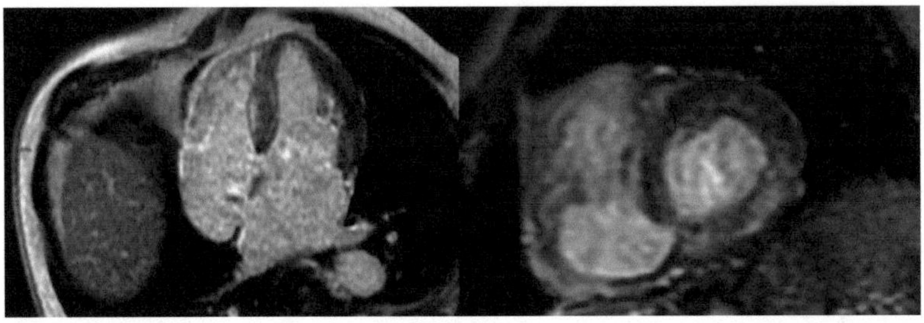

Figure 3.
Cardiovascular magnetic resonance imaging of myocardial late gadolinium enhancement with pronounced septal and basal distribution.

eliminated the difficulties of accurate TI selection, because tissue with the least gadolinium always appears nulled [50].

Krombach et al. described in 2007 another technic for the evaluation of CA using CMR [51]. The authors presented a measurement of myocardial T1 mapping values without application of LGE in identifying interstitial amyloid infiltration. Using this parameter, a sensitivity of 80% and a specificity of 94% was achieved in the study to diagnose CA. Determination of native and postcontrast (after application of the contrast agent) T1 mapping, allows for calculation of the extracellular volume (ECV), which correlates well with histological findings based on cardiac biopsies [52]. Meanwhile, several studies have demonstrated an increase in native T1 relaxation time as well as ECV of the myocardium in CA [53]. However, the diagnostic significance of ECV is limited due to overlap with other myocardial diseases associated with LV hypertrophy. Therefore, thresholds for native T1 relaxation time and ECV have not been established yet [54].

Due to the above-described comprehensive technical features, CMR represents an alternative to biopsy and has become an established part of the standard clinical pathway for CA diagnosis. In addition, it may provide prognostic information for patients with a confirmed diagnosis.

2.5 Cardiac scintigraphy

Tc-labeled cardiac scintigraphy provides incremental value to echocardiography and CMR, because of the ability to distinguish ATTR CA from other forms of LV hypertrophy [55]. Radionuclides have affinity towards myocardial amyloid deposits, especially towards myocardial ATTR. The binding of the radiotracer towards myocardial ATTR is supposed to be due to microcalcifications [56]. Three different technetium-labeled radiotracers are used for the diagnosis of ATTR-CA: ^{99}mTc-PYP (^{99}mTc-labeled pyrophosphate), ^{99}mTc-DPD (^{99}mTc-labeled 3,3- diphosphono-1,2-propanodicarboxylic acid), and ^{99}mTc-HMDP (^{99}mTc-labeled hydroxymethyl diphosphonate). Grading systems for the degree of uptake in the myocardium on planar imaging are quantitative and qualitative. Qualitative scores are based on the heart to contralateral lung uptake (H/CL) ratio with ^{99}mTc-PYP or the heart to whole body ratio with ^{99}mTc-DPD and ^{99}mTc-HDMP (**Figure 4**) [57].

Gillmore et al. assessed the diagnostic accuracy of all three above-mentioned tracers in 1,217 patients with suspected CA. Any myocardial radiotracer uptake was >99% sensitive and 86% specific for detecting ATTR-CA, with the majority of false-positive results from patients with AL-amyloidosis. A higher amount of myocardial radiotracer uptake (grade 2 or 3) and the absence of monoclonal proteins in serum or urine had nearly 100% specificity and 100% positive predictive value for ATTR-CA [55]. Imaging differentiation between AL and ATTR-amyloidosis

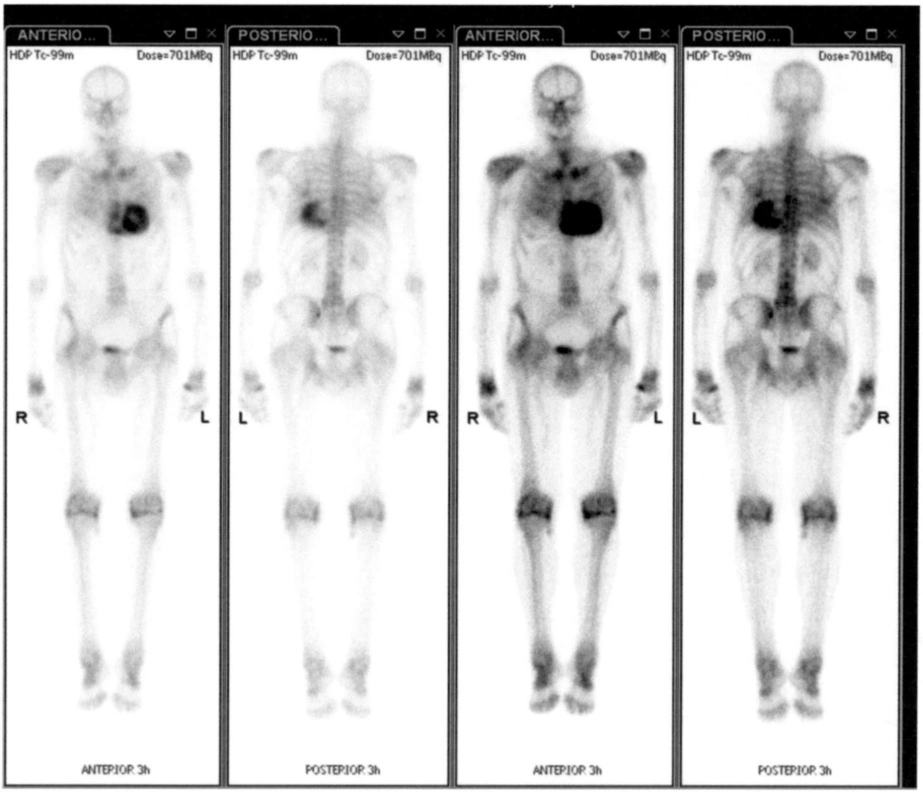

Figure 4.
99mTc-HMDP bone scintigraphy for diagnosis of cardiac amyloidosis.

is based on the ^{99}mTc-PYP H/CL uptake ratio; a ratio of <1.5 favors AL, whereas a ratio of ≥1.5 favors ATTR [58]. Semi-quantitative evaluation using ^{99}mTc-PYP planar imaging, a H/CL ratio of >1.5 at 1 h accurately distinguished ATTR from AL-CA with 97% sensitivity and 100% specificity and a whole-body retention of ^{99}mTc-DPD at 3 h is highly sensitive and specific for ATTR-CA [59].

In conclusion, Tc-labeled cardiac scintigraphy can reliably diagnose ATTR-amyloidosis in the absence of tissue biopsy, especially in cases of high myocardial radiotracer uptake and after laboratory exclusion of AL-amyloidosis.

3. Conclusion

Cardiac involvement in amyloidosis has a high mortality rate. For instance, patients with AL-amyloidosis have a 50% survival rate per year after the first episode of acute heart failure. Rapid diagnosis and initiation of chemotherapy are crucial in these patients. Besides, ATTR-amyloidosis may benefit from novel therapeutic options to improve symptoms and survival. The following features should raise the suspicion of CA: patients above 60 years of age with a low-flow low-gradient aortic stenosis, unexplained LV hypertrophy or peripheral sensory neuropathy, and patients with monoclonal gammopathy or elevated FLC levels. Non-invasive imaging technics are valuable in the assessment of CA and should be used widely. Cardiac imaging findings in echocardiography, CMR, or Tc-labeled bone or cardiac scintigraphy, are specific enough to diagnose CA in the setting of a positive non-cardiac biopsy (**Figure 5**). EMB with histological analysis of myocardial tissue is not essential anymore.

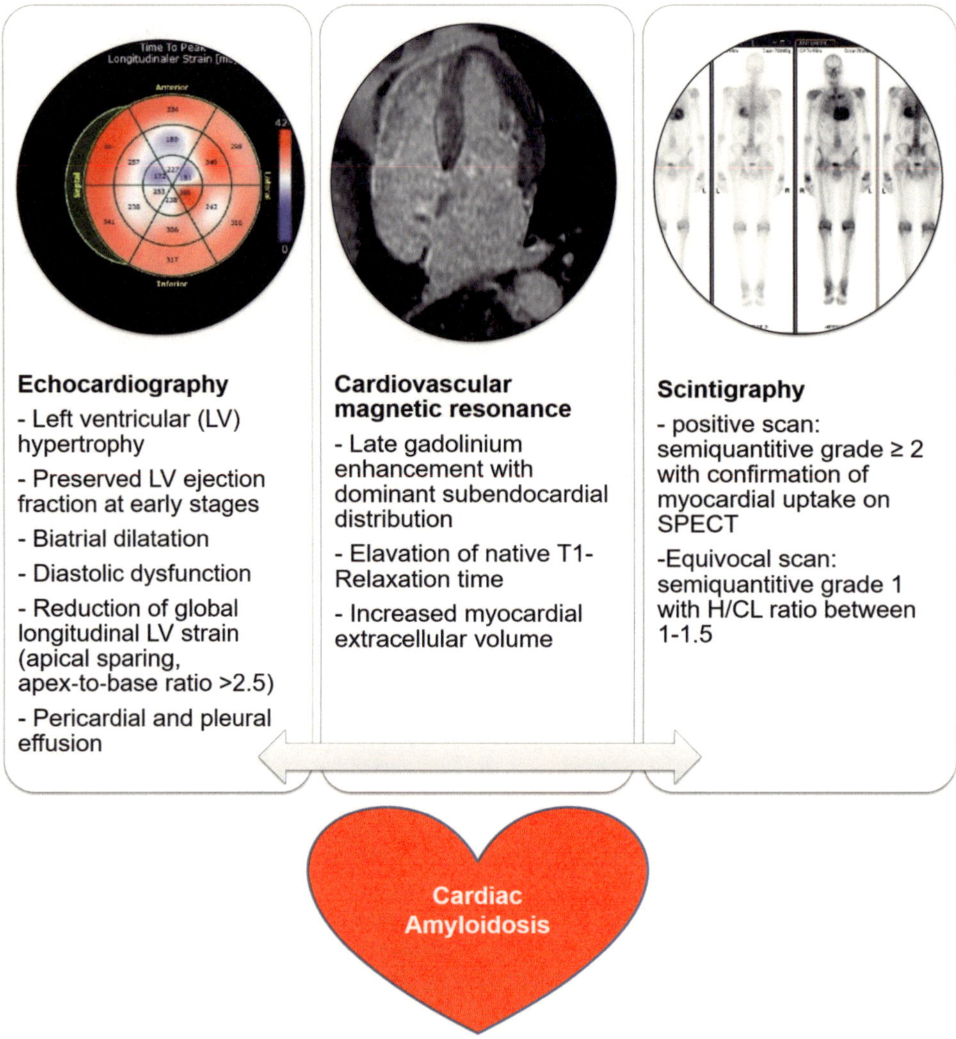

Figure 5.
Typical imaging features to diagnose cardiac amyloidosis.

Conflict of interest

NA and DZ has received meeting support from Pfizer. The other authors declare no conflict of interest.

Abbreviations

AL	Light chain amyloidosis
AMYLI	AMYLoidosis Index
ANF	Atrial natriuretic factor
ATTR	Amyloid transthyretin amyloidosis
ATTRm	Mutant transthyretin amyloidosis
ATTRwt	Transthyretin wild-type amyloidosis
AV	atrioventricular
BNP	Brain natriuretic peptide

CA	Cardiac amyloidosis
CMR	Cardiovacular magnetic resonance imaging
ECG	Electrocardiography
ECV	Extracellular volume
EMB	Endomyocardial biopsy
EPS	Electrophyisiology study
ESC	European Society of Cardiology
GLS	Global longitudinal strain
HCM	Hypertrophic cardiomyopathy
HV	His-ventricular
ICD	Implantable cardioverter defibrillator
LGE	Late gadolinium enhancement
LVEF	Left ventricular ejection fraction
NT-proBNP	N-terminal brain natriuretic peptide
PSIR	Phase-sensitive inversion recovery
RV	Right ventricular
SAA	Serum amyloid A
SCD	Sudden cardiac death
sFLC	Serum free light chain
SPECT	Single photon emission computed tomography
SSFP	Steady-state free precession
T4	Thyroid hormone thyroxine
TAVI	Transcatheter aortic valve implantation
Tc	technicium
TDI	Tissue Doppler imaging
TnI	Troponin I
TnT	Troponin T
TTR	Transthyretin
^{99}mTc-PYP	^{99}mTc-labeled pyrophosphate
^{99}mTc-DPD	^{99}mTc-labeled 3,3- diphosphono-1,2-propanodicarboxylic acid
^{99}mTc-HMDP	^{99}mTc-labeled hydroxymethyl diphosphonate

Author details

Eva Strickler, Ernest Tsiaze, Gerrit Hellige, Dominik Zumstein, Dominik Waldmeier and Nisha Arenja*
Kantonsspital Olten, Solothurner Spitäler AG, Olten, Switzerland

*Address all correspondence to: nisha.arenja@spital.so.ch

References

[1] J. D. Sipe *et al.*, "Nomenclature 2014: Amyloid fibril proteins and clinical classification of the amyloidosis," Amyloid. 2014, doi: 10.3109/13506129.2014.964858.

[2] G. Merlini *et al.*, "Systemic immunoglobulin light chain amyloidosis," *Nat. Rev. Dis. Prim.*, 2018, doi: 10.1038/s41572-018-0034-3.

[3] G. Merlini, D. C. Seldin, and M. A. Gertz, "Amyloidosis: Pathogenesis and new therapeutic options," *Journal of Clinical Oncology*. 2011, doi: 10.1200/JCO.2010.32.2271.

[4] K. Ablasser, N. Verheyen, T. Glantschnig, G. Agnetti, and P. P. Rainer, "Unfolding Cardiac Amyloidosis –From Pathophysiology to Cure," *Curr. Med. Chem.*, 2018, doi: 10.2174/0929867325666180104153338.

[5] H. H. Schmidt *et al.*, "Estimating the global prevalence of transthyretin familial amyloid polyneuropathy," *Muscle and Nerve*, 2018, doi: 10.1002/mus.26034.

[6] M. Grogan *et al.*, "Natural History of Wild-Type Transthyretin Cardiac Amyloidosis and Risk Stratification Using a Novel Staging System," *J. Am. Coll. Cardiol.*, 2016, doi: 10.1016/j.jacc.2016.06.033.

[7] F. Perfetto *et al.*, "The Val142Ile transthyretin cardiac amyloidosis: more than an Afro-American pathogenic variant," *J. Community Hosp. Intern. Med. Perspect.*, 2015, doi: 10.3402/jchimp.v5.26931.

[8] F. Cappelli *et al.*, "The Val142Ile transthyretin cardiac amyloidosis: Not only an Afro-American pathogenic variant? A single-centre Italian experience," *J. Cardiovasc. Med.*, 2016, doi: 10.2459/JCM.0000000000000290.

[9] M. Tanskanen *et al.*, "Senile systemic amyloidosis affects 25% of the very aged and associates with genetic variation in alpha2-macroglobulin and tau: A population-based autopsy study," *Ann. Med.*, 2008, doi: 10.1080/07853890701842988.

[10] P. P. Liu and D. Smyth, "Wild-Type Transthyretin Amyloid Cardiomyopathy: A Missed Cause of Heart Failure with Preserved Ejection Fraction with Evolving Treatment Implications," *Circulation*. 2016, doi: 10.1161/CIRCULATIONAHA.115.020351.

[11] P. R. Scully *et al.*, "Prevalence of Cardiac Amyloidosis in Patients Referred for Transcatheter Aortic Valve Replacement," *Journal of the American College of Cardiology*. 2018, doi: 10.1016/j.jacc.2017.11.037.

[12] J. Ternacle *et al.*, "Aortic Stenosis and Cardiac Amyloidosis: JACC Review Topic of the Week," *Journal of the American College of Cardiology*. 2019, doi: 10.1016/j.jacc.2019.09.056.

[13] E. González-López *et al.*, "Clinical characteristics of wild-type transthyretin cardiac amyloidosis: Disproving myths," *Eur. Heart J.*, 2017, doi: 10.1093/eurheartj/ehx043.

[14] C. Röcken and A. Shakespeare, "Pathology, diagnosis and pathogenesis of AA amyloidosis," *Virchows Archiv*. 2002, doi: 10.1007/s00428-001-0582-9.

[15] T. V. Kourelis *et al.*, "Presentation and Outcomes of Localized Immunoglobulin Light Chain Amyloidosis: The Mayo Clinic Experience," *Mayo Clin. Proc.*, 2017, doi: 10.1016/j.mayocp.2017.02.016.

[16] J. Guan, S. Mishra, R. H. Falk, and R. Liao, "Current perspectives on cardiac amyloidosis," *American Journal*

of Physiology - Heart and Circulatory Physiology. 2012, doi: 10.1152/ajpheart.00815.2011

[17] Singh V, Mendirichaga R, Savani GT, Rodriguez A, Blumer V, Elmariah S, Inglessis-Azuaje I, Palacios I. Comparison of Utilization Trends, Indications, and Complications of Endomyocardial Biopsy in Native Versus Donor Hearts (from the Nationwide Inpatient Sample 2002 to 2014). Am J Cardiol. 2018 Feb 1;121(3):356-363. doi: 10.1016/j.amjcard.2017.10.021.

[18] Yilmaz A, Kindermann I, Kindermann M, Mahfoud F, Ukena C, Athanasiadis A, Hill S, Mahrholdt H, Voehringer M, Schieber M, Klingel K, Kandolf R, Böhm M, Sechtem U. Comparative evaluation of left and right ventricular endomyocardial biopsy: differences in complication rate and diagnostic performance. Circulation. 2010 Aug 31;122(9):900-909. doi: 10.1161/CIRCULATIONAHA.109.924167.

[19] Chimenti C, Frustaci A. Contribution and risks of left ventricular endomyocardial biopsy in patients with cardiomyopathies: a retrospective study over a 28-year period. Circulation. 2013 Oct 1;128(14):1531-1541. doi: 10.1161/CIRCULATIONAHA.13.001414.

[20] Bennett MK, Gilotra NA, Harrington C, Rao S, Dunn JM, Freitag TB, Halushka MK, Russell SD. Evaluation of the role of endomyocardial biopsy in 851 patients with unexplained heart failure from 2000-2009. Circ Heart Fail. 2013 Jul;6(4):676-684. doi: 10.1161/CIRCHEARTFAILURE.112.000087.

[21] G. B. Hannibal, "Interpretation of the low-voltage ECG," *AACN Adv. Crit. Care*, 2014, doi: 10.1097/NCI.0000000000000001.

[22] C. Rapezzi *et al.*, "Systemic cardiac amyloidoses: Disease profiles and clinical courses of the 3 main types," *Circulation*, 2009, doi: 10.1161/CIRCULATIONAHA.108.843334.

[23] M. Boldrini *et al.*, "Prevalence and prognostic value of conduction disturbances at the time of diagnosis of cardiac AL amyloidosis," *Ann. Noninvasive Electrocardiol.*, 2013, doi: 10.1111/anec.12032.

[24] Z. Cheng, K. Zhu, Z. Tian, D. Zhao, Q. Cui, and Q. Fang, "The findings of electrocardiography in patients with cardiac amyloidosis," *Ann. Noninvasive Electrocardiol.*, 2013, doi: 10.1111/anec.12018.

[25] B. W. Sperry *et al.*, "Are classic predictors of voltage valid in cardiac amyloidosis? A contemporary analysis of electrocardiographic findings," *Int. J. Cardiol.*, 2016, doi: 10.1016/j.ijcard.2016.04.030.

[26] K. Sanchis *et al.*, "Atrial fibrillation and subtype of atrial fibrillation in cardiac amyloidosis: clinical and echocardiographic features, impact on mortality," *Amyloid*, 2019, doi: 10.1080/13506129.2019.1620724.

[27] M. Auer-Grumbach *et al.*, "Hereditary ATTR Amyloidosis in Austria: Prevalence and Epidemiological Hot Spots," *J. Clin. Med.*, 2020, doi: 10.3390/jcm9072234.

[28] D. K. Dawson *et al.*, "Prognostic role of CMR in patients presenting with ventricular arrhythmias," *JACC Cardiovasc. Imaging*, 2013, doi: 10.1016/j.jcmg.2012.09.012.

[29] J. Reisinger, S. W. Dubrey, M. Lavalley, M. Skinner, and R. H. Falk, "Electrophysiologic abnormalities in AL (primary) amyloidosis with cardiac involvement," *J. Am. Coll. Cardiol.*, 1997, doi: 10.1016/S0735-1097(97)00267-2.

[30] M. Orini *et al.*, "Noninvasive Mapping of the Electrophysiological

Substrate in Cardiac Amyloidosis and Its Relationship to Structural Abnormalities," *J. Am. Heart Assoc.*, 2019, doi: 10.1161/JAHA.119.012097.

[31] M. Brignole *et al.*, "2013 ESC Guidelines on cardiac pacing and cardiac resynchronization therapy: The Task Force on cardiac pacing and resynchronization therapy of the European Society of Cardiology (ESC). Developed in collaboration with the European Heart Rhythm Association," *Europace*, 2013, doi: 10.1093/europace/eut206.

[32] A. V. Kristen *et al.*, "Prophylactic implantation of cardioverter-defibrillator in patients with severe cardiac amyloidosis and high risk for sudden cardiac death," *Hear. Rhythm*, 2008, doi: 10.1016/j.hrthm.2007.10.016.

[33] E. P. Hess and R. D. White, "Out-of-hospital cardiac arrest in patients with cardiac amyloidosis: Presenting rhythms, management and outcomes in four patients," *Resuscitation*, 2004, doi: 10.1016/j.resuscitation.2003.08.007.

[34] S. G. Priori *et al.*, "2015 ESC Guidelines for the management of patients with ventricular arrhythmias and the prevention of sudden cardiac death: The Task Force for the Management of Patients with Ventricular Arrhythmias and the Prevention of Sudden Cardiac Death of the Europe," *Europace*, 2015, doi: 10.1093/europace/euv319.

[35] M. A. Gertz *et al.*, "Definition of organ involvement and treatment response in immunoglobulin light chain amyloidosis (AL): A consensus opinion from the 10th International Symposium on Amyloid and Amyloidosis," 2005, doi: 10.1002/ajh.20381.

[36] S. Kumar *et al.*, "Revised prognostic staging system for light chain amyloidosis incorporating cardiac biomarkers and serum free light chain measurements," *J. Clin. Oncol.*, 2012, doi: 10.1200/JCO.2011.38.5724.

[37] S. F. Nagueh *et al.*, "Recommendations for the evaluation of left ventricular diastolic function by echocardiography: An update from the American society of echocardiography and the European association of cardiovascular imaging," *Eur. Heart J. Cardiovasc. Imaging*, 2016, doi: 10.1093/ehjci/jew082.

[38] P. Elliott *et al.*, "Classification of the cardiomyopathies: A position statement from the european society of cardiology working group on myocardial and pericardial diseases," *Eur. Heart J.*, 2008, doi: 10.1093/eurheartj/ehm342.

[39] A. Aimo *et al.*, "A simple echocardiographic score to rule out cardiac amyloidosis," *Eur. J. Clin. Invest.*, 2020, doi: 10.1111/eci.13449.

[40] E. D. Pagourelias *et al.*, "Echo Parameters for Differential Diagnosis in Cardiac Amyloidosis: A Head-to-Head Comparison of Deformation and Nondeformation Parameters," *Circ. Cardiovasc. Imaging*, 2017, doi: 10.1161/CIRCIMAGING.116.005588.

[41] M. Boldrini *et al.*, "Multiparametric Echocardiography Scores for the Diagnosis of Cardiac Amyloidosis," *JACC Cardiovasc. Imaging*, 2020, doi: 10.1016/j.jcmg.2019.10.011.

[42] G. Y. Lee *et al.*, "Visual assessment of relative apical sparing pattern is more useful than quantitative assessment for diagnosing cardiac amyloidosis in borderline or mildly increased left ventricular wall thickness," *Circ. J.*, 2015, doi: 10.1253/circj.CJ-14-1328.

[43] S. J. Buss *et al.*, "Longitudinal left ventricular function for prediction of survival in systemic light-chain amyloidosis: Incremental value compared with clinical and biochemical markers," *J. Am. Coll. Cardiol.*, 2012, doi: 10.1016/j.jacc.2012.04.043.

[44] S. Arvidsson, M. Y. Henein, G. Wikström, O. B. Suhr, and P. Lindqvist, "Right ventricular involvement in transthyretin amyloidosis," *Amyloid*, 2018, doi: 10.1080/13506129.2018.1493989.

[45] Khor YM, Cuddy S, Falk RH, Dorbala S. Multimodality Imaging in the Evaluation and Management of Cardiac Amyloidosis. Semin Nucl Med. 2020 Jul;50(4):295-310. doi: 10.1053/j.semnuclmed.2020.01.001. Epub 2020 Feb 9. PMID: 32540027.

[46] M. Fontana, "Prognosis in Cardiac Amyloidosis by LGE: Ready for Prime Time?∗," *JACC: Cardiovascular Imaging*. 2016, doi: 10.1016/j.jcmg.2015.11.028.

[47] M. Yazaki *et al.*, "Cardiac amyloid in patients with familial amyloid polyneuropathy consists of abundant wild-type transthyretin," *Biochem. Biophys. Res. Commun.*, 2000, doi: 10.1006/bbrc.2000.3203.

[48] A. M. Maceira *et al.*, "Cardiovascular magnetic resonance in cardiac amyloidosis," *Circulation*, 2005, doi: 10.1161/01.CIR.0000152819.97857.9D.

[49] M. Fontana *et al.*, "Prognostic value of late gadolinium enhancement cardiovascular magnetic resonance in cardiac amyloidosis," *Circulation*, 2015, doi: 10.1161/CIRCULATIONAHA.115.016567.

[50] T. Pandey, K. Jambhekar, R. Shaikh, S. Lensing, and S. Viswamitra, "Utility of the inversion scout sequence (TI scout) in diagnosing myocardial amyloid infiltration," *Int. J. Cardiovasc. Imaging*, 2013, doi: 10.1007/s10554-012-0042-4.

[51] G. A. Krombach *et al.*, "Cardiac amyloidosis: MR imaging findings and T1 quantification, comparison with control subjects," J. Magn. Reson. Imaging, 2007, doi: 10.1002/jmri.20917.

[52] T. D. Karamitsos *et al.*, "Noncontrast T1 mapping for the diagnosis of cardiac amyloidosis," *JACC Cardiovasc. Imaging*, 2013, doi: 10.1016/j.jcmg.2012.11.013.

[53] A. Martinez-Naharro *et al.*, "Native T1 and Extracellular Volume in Transthyretin Amyloidosis," *JACC Cardiovasc. Imaging*, 2019, doi: 10.1016/j.jcmg.2018.02.006.

[54] D. R. Messroghli *et al.*, "Clinical recommendations for cardiovascular magnetic resonance mapping of T1, T2, T2 and extracellular volume: A consensus statement by the Society for Cardiovascular Magnetic Resonance (SCMR) endorsed by the European Association for Cardiovascular Imagin," *Journal of Cardiovascular Magnetic Resonance*. 2017, doi: 10.1186/s12968-017-0389-8.

[55] J. D. Gillmore *et al.*, "Nonbiopsy diagnosis of cardiac transthyretin amyloidosis," *Circulation*, 2016, doi: 10.1161/CIRCULATIONAHA.116.021612.

[56] M. A. Stats and J. R. Stone, "Varying levels of small microcalcifications and macrophages in ATTR and AL cardiac amyloidosis: implications for utilizing nuclear medicine studies to subtype amyloidosis," *Cardiovasc. Pathol.*, 2016, doi: 10.1016/j.carpath.2016.07.001.

[57] S. Dorbala *et al.*, "ASNC/AHA/ASE/EANM/HFSA/ISA/SCMR/SNMMI expert consensus recommendations for multimodality imaging in cardiac amyloidosis: Part 1 of 2—evidence base and standardized methods of imaging," *J. Nucl. Cardiol.*, 2019, doi: 10.1007/s12350-019-01760-6.

[58] Y. J. Kim, S. Ha, and Y. il Kim, "Cardiac amyloidosis imaging with amyloid positron emission tomography: A systematic review and meta-analysis," *J. Nucl. Cardiol.*, 2020, doi: 10.1007/s12350-018-1365-x.

[59] E. Perugini *et al.*, "Noninvasive etiologic diagnosis of cardiac amyloidosis using 99mTc-3,3-diphosphono-1,2-propanodicarboxylic acid scintigraphy," *J. Am. Coll. Cardiol.*, 2005, doi: 10.1016/j.jacc.2005.05.073.

Chapter 5

A Short Review of Hematopoietic Transplantation for AL Amyloidosis

Ivetta Danylesko

Abstract

AL amyloidosis is an uncommon disease with variable clinical presentations; as such, it is often initially unrecognized and diagnosis is therefore frequently delayed. As a result of diagnosis at a point in their disease when patients often have significant end-organ damage, aggressive therapy with major toxicities can be extremely challenging. Nonetheless, clinical data have been accumulating over the past several decades that have demonstrated that patients who were taken to high-dose therapy—typically using single-agent L-phenylalanine mustard—with autologous hematopoietic rescue, have a dramatically improved overall survival than otherwise. In this chapter, the critical clinical data that demonstrate this, and the risk-adjusted approach to optimize the outcome for patients, are reviewed.

Keywords: AL amyloidosis, hematopoietic transplant, plasma cell dyscrasias

1. Introduction

AL amyloidosis, the consequence of the three-dimensional misfolding and aggregation of serum immunoglobulin light chains, with consequent end-organ damage due to the deposition of the amyloid, is an uncommon disorder, resulting from a clonal proliferation of lymphoid cells of B cell lineage. As such, it shares many pathobiological characteristics with multiple myeloma, and drugs that have antineoplastic activity in myeloma and other plasma cell dyscrasias typically are active in the treatment of AL amyloidosis. However, in large part, because the early clinical manifestations of AL amyloidosis can be insidious and nonspecific, a majority of patients with AL amyloidosis are not diagnosed until there has been significant end-organ damage. The presence of end-organ damage, often in multiple organ systems critical for the tolerance of antineoplastic therapy, has limited the feasible treatment options for patients with significant amyloid burden, particularly with regard to cardiac, hepatic, and renal involvement by amyloid.

Despite the barriers to treatment, however, significant progress has been made, especially at centers with deep experience in the management of AL amyloidosis. Clinical data have been accumulated in the past several decades that convincingly demonstrates—despite little in the way of prospective, randomized trials—that high-dose antineoplastic therapy with hematopoietic rescue, and most specifically high-dose melphalan chemotherapy with autologous stem cell rescue—"ABMT," improves overall survival in patients with AL amyloidosis. As of this writing, criteria for selecting patients for ABMT are evolving, as risk stratification becomes better defined, and supportive care improves. For patients who are considered for transplant, these factors also impact the decision as to whether a particular patient is an appropriate candidate for upfront ABMT, versus induction therapy followed by ABMT. Similarly, post-transplant maintenance therapy is also the subject of ongoing clinical research. This review summarizes the data from a number of important papers published in the peer-reviewed medical literature, all of which are indexed in the National Library of Medicine of the United States' searchable database, PubMed.

2. Evolution of transplant for AL amyloidosis

The historical evolution of the treatment of AL amyloidosis is reviewed elsewhere in this volume. The first peer-reviewed report of the efficacy of conventional doses of L-phenylalanine mustard—melphalan—dates to 1958, when Blokhin and colleagues in the former Soviet Union reported benefit from the use of melphalan in a variety of disease states [1]. Shortly thereafter, in 1962, Mass reported some degree of efficacy of prednisone as a single agent in the treatment of myeloma, as compared to placebo [2]. However, it was not until 1997 that the efficacy of melphalan and prednisone for the treatment of AL amyloidosis was reported in the context of a formal clinical trial. In that year, Kyle and colleagues at the Mayo Clinic reported the results of a prospective, randomized clinical trial, comparing colchicine alone, melphalan together with prednisone, or the combination of all three drugs, in treating AL amyloidosis. That study randomized 220 patients who had biopsy documentation of AL amyloidosis. The authors reported median survival of 18 months for patients randomized to melphalan and prednisone, the median survival of 17 months for patients randomized to the three-drug combination, and median survival of 8.5 months for those treated using colchicine alone [3]. This study established melphalan with prednisone as a standard of care, although this approach had by then been in use for more than two decades.

ABMT for patients with amyloidosis began to be explored extensively in the final decade of the twentieth century at a number of centers around the world. In 1996, in the journal Blood, Comenzo and colleagues at Boston City Hospital reported their experience with their first five AL amyloidosis patients treated using intravenous melphalan at a dose of 100 mg/meter square body surface area per day for two consecutive days, followed by rescue with autologous peripheral blood hematopoietic progenitor cells that were collected after filgrastim priming [4]. Patients underwent this therapy between 2 and 18 months after diagnosis, with a median of transplant at 5 months from diagnosis; median age was 46 years. All five patients were alive at the time of publishing follow up, with favorable hematologic responses—clearing of monoclonal light chains, and clinical improvements with respect to their manifestations of disease, including peripheral neuropathy in the three patients so affected, gastrointestinal dysfunction in the one patient so affected, and resolution of hepatomegaly in the one patient so affected. Performance status either was improved or stable for all five patients. Similarly, Moreau reported a retrospective examination of a series of 21 patients with AL amyloidosis treated in France, published in 1998 [5]. In this series, 18 patients received single-agent high-dose melphalan, in the range of 200 mg/meter square body surface area, and three patients received the combination of high-dose melphalan together with total body radiation. Up to 43% of these patients died within the first month after transplant, an extremely high mortality rate attributable to toxicity, as opposed to the progression of the disease. However, among the surviving

12 patients in this series, 10 patients had an objective response to therapy, demonstrating that the therapy did have efficacy for those who tolerated the treatment. Overall survival was 57% at a median follow up of 14 months, and Event-free survival was 29.9% [4]. Importantly, they noted five clinical features at the time of transplant that was associated with outcome. Patient results were significantly worse if there was (a) greater than 3 grams per 24 hours' proteinuria; (b) creatinine clearance less than 30 mL/minute; (c) congestive heart failure syndrome; (d) neuropathy; or (e) hepatomegaly together with alkaline phosphatase greater than 200. As would be expected, patients with two or more of these adverse clinical findings had significantly poorer outcomes, with overall survival at 4 years of 11.1%, as compared to the overall survival of 91.7% for patients with fewer than two of these adverse findings.

Reports such as those by Comenzo and Moreau, and from a number of other centers around the world regarding the early experiences with autologous transplant for treatment of AL amyloidosis, led the Intergroupe Francophone du Myelome (IFM) to conduct a prospective, randomized multicenter clinical trial, comparing high-dose melphalan with autologous hematopoietic rescue—ABMT—to conventional-dose melphalan given with dexamethasone. The findings from this study were reported by Jaccard and colleagues on behalf of the IFM in the year 2007 [6]. Between the years 2000 and 2005, 100 patients were accrued who had Eastern Cooperative Oncology Group performance status score of 2 or lower, with biopsy-proven AL amyloidosis, in the absence of symptomatic multiple myeloma. In the transplant group, peripheral blood hematopoietic progenitor cells were collected by cytapheresis following a five-day course of granulocyte-colony stimulating factor, with a minimum target collection of 2 million CD34 cells per kg body weight. Conditioning was with melphalan 200 mg/meter square but was reduced to 140 mg/meter square for patients 65 years of age and older, for those with left ventricular cardiac ejection fraction less than 30%, those with calculated creatinine clearance less than 30 mL per minute, and those with liver disease who had significantly prolonged prothrombin time, elevated total bilirubin greater than five times the upper limit of normal, or alkaline phosphatase elevated to greater than five times upper limit of normal. The granulocyte-colony stimulating factor was administered to accelerate granulocyte recovery following stem cell infusion. Patients in the control arm were treated using monthly cycles of oral melphalan 10 mg per meter square body surface area on days 1–4 each month, together with oral dexamethasone 40 mg daily for days 1–4 each month, for up to 18 months, later emended to stop therapy after 12 months if complete remission obtained. Dose adjustments were permitted for oral melphalan if clinically appropriate. In this study, criteria for organ involvement and organ response were meticulously defined. The two cohorts were fairly well balanced for age, performance status, the number of organs clinically involved by disease, and organ function.

Among the 50 subjects randomized to the ABMT arm, 13 did not proceed to transplant, of whom 10 died from complications of the amyloidosis prior to transplant. Of the 37 patients who did proceed to ABMT, nine died within 100 days of receiving the melphalan conditioning; transplant-related mortality was 24%. Among the patients assigned to conventional-dose melphalan, two patients died from cardiac arrhythmias prior to completing the first month of therapy, and five additional patients died within the first 130 days after randomization—all from the progression of the underlying amyloid disease. The results reported showed that hematologic responses did not differ significantly between the two treatment groups. Up to 69% of the patients in the conventional-dose therapy group demonstrated favorable reductions in light chain levels, as compared to 62% in the transplant arm. However, the complete remission rate was 47% in the conventional-dose group, as compared to 61% in the high-dose melphalan group. As of the time of data analysis in August 2006, 51 patients had died out of the initial 100, 20 patients in the conventional-dose group, and 31 patients in the group assigned to transplant. With respect to intention-to-treat analysis, the estimated median overall survival was 56.9 months in the conventional dose cohort, as compared to 22.2 months in the group assigned to ABMT. The study was powered to detect at 25% survival advantage for ABMT as compared to conventional-dose melphalan with dexamethasone; the study failed to demonstrate the superiority of ABMT. Indeed, in this study, median overall survival was significantly longer in the conventional-dose control group, as compared to the autologous transplant group. The authors noted that had the trial been conducted exclusively at a tertiary referral center with a very high level of expertise, the mortality in the transplant arm might have been lower. This study did appear to have a somewhat chilling effect on enthusiasm for high-dose therapy with the autologous hematopoietic rescue for the treatment of AL amyloidosis for a brief period of time, but centers with experience continued to investigate this approach, particularly as supportive care improved and the experience was gained.

As clinical experience accrued, demonstrating that end-organ function at the time of transplant largely determined early survival during and shortly after the transplant, along with the observation that patients who survived the acute toxicities of transplant showed a very high likelihood of a favorable response, it became clear that selecting appropriate patients for transplant based on organ function, performance status, and risk stratification was essential to optimize outcome from high-dose therapy. Over the past 25 years, the application of risk stratification to patient selection for transplant has translated into decreased acute mortality in published reports of ABMT for AL amyloidosis. Gertz and colleagues published a consensus opinion on the definition of organ involvement and treatment response in AL amyloidosis from the 10th international symposium on amyloid and amyloidosis [7], in 2005. The investigators who participated in writing this report carefully specified criteria for the diagnosis of AL amyloid—as distinct from other potential diagnoses, such as myeloma. They also specified the formal definition of specific organ involvement—for most organs by biopsy documentation but for some organs noninvasive findings (e.g., for definitive lung involvement, classic diffuse interstitial lung disease on CT imaging together with biopsy-proven AL amyloidosis in a different organ). Further, they defined criteria for evaluating treatment response by organ, including definitions of complete response, partial response, stable disease, and progression of the disease. The rigorous application of these types of definitions helped to harmonize patient assessment in the context of data reporting, and analysis of patient responses to ABMT as well as conventional therapies and investigational agents. Formalizing the criteria for diagnosis, organ involvement, and response to treatment, in turn, enhanced the analysis of risk stratification of patients.

Many of the prominent early series of patients with AL amyloidosis treated by ABMT were reviewed in a paper published by Comenzo and Gertz, two leaders in Amyloidosis research and treatment, in the journal Blood in the year 2002 [7]. These authors summarized from four single-center clinical trials, totaling 87 patients, and from two multicenter reports, totaling 61 patients. Among the 87 patients reported from the four single-center experiences, transplant-related mortality (TRM) was 16 patients, a rate of 21% at that time. A summation of responses for the four single-center series was a 62% response rate overall. In the two multicenter series summarized by Comenzo and Gertz (Table 1 in their manuscript) TRM was measured as 24 patients out of 61 subjects, for transplant-related mortality of 39% in these two reports, and with overall response rate reported also at 62%.

During the first two decades of the twenty-first century, increasing numbers of centers reported their experiences with a series of AL amyloidosis patients undergoing ABMT, and with increased experience, as well as more refined selection criteria were applied, transplant-related mortality fell over time.

In 2015, D'Souza and her colleagues published an important summary of data compiled by the Center for International Blood and Marrow Transplant Research (CIBMTR) regarding the outcome for autologous transplantation to treat AL amyloidosis. This report analyzed data from 1536 patients with a diagnosis of AL amyloidosis who underwent ABMT at 134 transplant centers between the years 1995 and 2012, as entered into the CIBMTR database [8]. Data from these patients were grouped into three chronologic cohorts—the group of patients transplanted between the years 1995 and 2000; patients transplanted between the years 2001 and 2006; and finally, patients transplanted between the years 2007 and 2012. The median age at transplantation was 56 for the cohort as a whole, with the median age gradually rising in successive chronologic cohorts, with most patients undergoing autologous transplants within 6 months of diagnosis. The underlying plasma cell clone was lambda in 72% of transplant patients. The median melphalan dose was 175 mg/meter square body surface area for the cohort transplanted between 2001 to 2006 but fell to 143 mg/m2 body surface area during 2007–2012. The percentage of patients that received antineoplastic therapy prior to transplant was 85% between 2001 and 2006, but the percentage of patients receiving antineoplastic therapy prior to transplant fell to 67% for those transplanted between 2007 and 2012. Early mortality—that is, death by day 30 and by day 100, declined significantly over time. Mortality by day 30 was 11%, and mortality by day 100 was 20%, in the patients transplanted between 1995 and 2000. However, mortality by day 30 fell to 3%, and mortality by day 100 fell to 5%, for the cohort transplanted between the years 2007 and 2012. Consistent with the improved outcome associated with decreased early mortality from transplant over time, overall survival also improved substantially over time. Five-year overall survival was 55% in the cohort of patients transplanted between the years 1995 and 2000. This improved to a 5-year survival of 77% for the cohort transplanted between the years 2007 and 2012. In their discussion, the authors of this paper attributed improvements in outcome both to improvements in supportive care, as well as increasing clinical expertise at managing patients through the transplant process. They also remarked that the best results for ABMT in AL amyloidosis as of that writing came from high-volume transplant centers, and noted that in the data set analyzed, ABMT centers performing fewer than four transplants per year for treatment of AL amyloidosis had higher early mortality rates than centers that performed a number greater than four transplants per year. Multivariate analysis in this study indicated that the presence of cardiac involvement, the presence of poor renal function, the presence of poor performance status (Karnofsky performance status of less than 80%), and use of melphalan conditioning at a dose of less than 180 mg/meter square body surface area—were all associated with worse outcome. **Figure 1** illustrates an approximation of the Kaplan–Meier survival curves for patients in the analysis of the CIBMTR data referenced above.

The conditioning regimen that has become standard over the past quarter-century for myeloma patients undergoing autologous transplant is melphalan as a single agent, at 200 mg/meter square body surface area, given either as a single dose, or divided over 2 consecutive days. Tandon and colleagues from the Mayo Clinic examined their experience with making adjustments to the melphalan dose [9]. In this retrospective analysis of 457 patients, 314 of these—69%—received full-intensity therapy with melphalan given at 200 mg/meter square. Up to 143 patients, that is, 31%, were treated using reduced-intensity therapy, defined as less

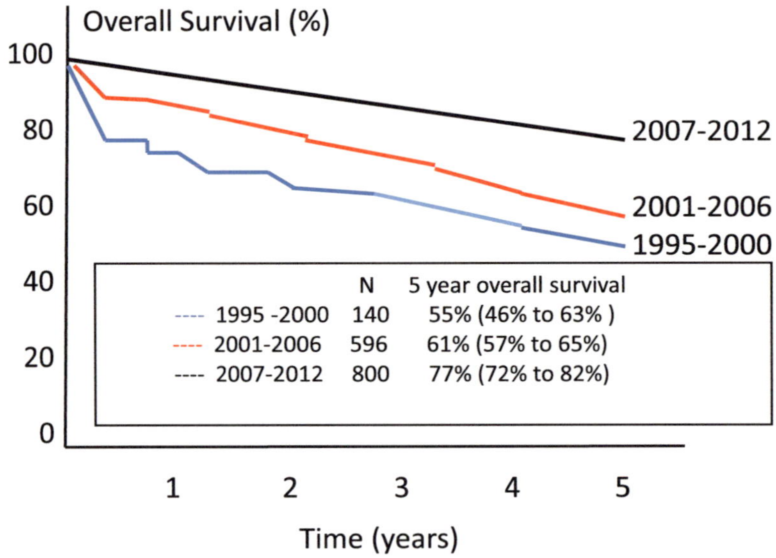

Figure 1.
Probability of overall survival after autologous transplantation in AL amyloidosis for three different time periods: European bone marrow transplant registry data (after D'Souzaetal, J clinical oncology 2015 [8]).

than 180 mg/meter square; most often, the reduced dose cohort were treated using melphalan at 140 mg/meter square. The authors stated that the conditioning dose of melphalan was adjusted depending on performance status, the patient's comorbidities, and the presence of renal insufficiency, defined as serum creatinine greater than or equal to 2 mg/dL. In their analysis, patients who received full-intensity therapy were, as expected, overall younger, with better average performance status, and with less multi-organ involvement by amyloidosis and, in especial, less cardiac disease, than patients who received dose reduced melphalan. Progression-free survival was significantly longer in the full-intensity therapy group as compared to the reduced-intensity therapy group, with four-year progression-free survival of 55% for those receiving full-dose therapy, as compared to 31% for those receiving dose reduced melphalan. Overall survival was also significantly longer, reported as 86% overall survival at 4 years for the patients receiving full intensity melphalan, as compared to 54% overall survival at 4 years for the patients who received dose reduced melphalan. To date, there has been relatively little investigation into alternative conditioning regimens. Sanchorawala and colleagues from Boston did report a small pilot study in which bortezomib at a dose of 1 mg/meter square on days minus 6, minus 3, plus 1, and plus 4, was added to the conditioning regimen of melphalan. In this study, melphalan was given at either 200 mg/meter square divided over 2 days—for 8 patients, and melphalan was given at 140 mg/meter square divided over 2 days for 1 patient who was aged over 65. Hematologic responses were achieved in 89% of the patients, with no toxic deaths [10]. No long-term follow-up data were provided. This approach has not been adopted in general, and indeed, single-agent melphalan at 200 mg/meter square remains the conventional dose applied to patients for conditioning in the setting of ABMT for AL amyloidosis.

Allogeneic hematopoietic transplantation has very rarely been performed as therapy of systemic AL amyloidosis [11, 12]. The majority of patients with AL amyloidosis have a low plasma cell burden. Further, there is a very low risk of contamination of peripheral blood hematopoietic progenitor cells by the malignant plasma cell clone. Finally, there is a significantly greater risk of severe complications from allogeneic as compared to autologous transplant. On the basis of these considerations, allogeneic hematopoietic transplant continues to be applied rarely to the management of systemic AL amyloidosis.

3. Evolution of risk stratification

Clinical prognosis at any point in time for a patient diagnosed with AL amyloidosis correlates, on the one hand, with the biological features of the clone of cells producing the pathogenic immunoglobulin light chain, and, on the other hand, with the damage to the end organs that has resulted from the amyloid deposition. Although the characteristics of the abnormal clone (most often a plasma cell but in a minority of cases a B cell giving rise to an IgM-associated light chain) may correlate with parameters of end-organ damage, it tends to be the measures of end-organ damage that impact the most on risk stratification useful for assessing patients' risk of morbidity and mortality at ABMT. Dittrich and colleagues, from Heidelberg, Germany, recently reviewed the prognosis and staging of AL amyloidosis [13]. Adverse features of the underlying plasma cell clone that are particularly statistically significant include bone marrow plasmacytosis greater than 10% morphologically, and elevation of the involved free light chain, greater than 125 mg/liter in the plasma, especially when greater than 180 mg/liter [14]. Chromosomal abnormalities identified by karyotype or by fluorescent *in situ* hybridization are also of prognostic significance [15].

However, with respect to risk for transplant-related morbidity and mortality, biomarkers of end-organ damage are particularly important to assessing patients as candidates for high-dose therapy. Numerous organ features and biomarkers have been examined, but the most prominent markers relate to cardiac function and renal function, with hepatic and pulmonary function, as well as nutritional status, also becoming important if impaired. The Mayo Clinic group published a cardiac staging system for AL amyloidosis patients in 2004, using the two parameters of (a) elevated circulating serum troponin level as a measure of myocardial cell damage, and (b) elevated N-terminal pro-B type natriuretic peptide (NT-proBNP) level [16]. In this system, patients with high-sensitivity troponin levels greater than 54 pg./microliter, or NT-proBNP greater than 332 ng/liter, but not both, were categorized as stage I, with a median survival of 130 months. Patients with troponin level and NT-proBNP above both thresholds were categorized as Stage III disease and had a median survival of only 10 months. In 2012, the Mayo Clinic group revised their system to expand the grouping to four stages [17], in the process of raising the threshold for the NT-proBNP to greater than 1800 ng/liter and adding the criterion of the difference between the involved free light chain and the uninvolved free light chain (termed d FLC) being greater than 180 mg/liter being an adverse prognostic factor. In this staging system, patients with all the adverse factors—stage IV disease—had a median overall survival of only 6 months; those with only the two cardiac adverse parameters had stage III disease with median overall survival of 24 months. Since then, additional staging systems have been proposed for assessing cardiac status, but are variations on the Mayo approach. One means of addressing severe cardiac disease due to amyloid infiltration has been to take selected patients to heart transplantation, and, upon recovery, follow heart transplantation by ABMT. Less dramatic approaches that have been widely applied have included, where appropriate, pre-ABMT implantation of an automated cardiac defibrillator, and use of ventricular support devices in severe heart failure that is expected to improve after ABMT. Cardiac support in patients with AL amyloidosis was recently reviewed in detail by Macedo and colleagues from Brazil [18].

Similarly, staging systems to categorize renal end-organ damage in AL amyloidosis have been developed. Kastritis and colleagues published a staging system for renal disease in this setting [19] using the ratio of 24-hour proteinuria (24-hour UPr) to estimate glomerular filtration rate (e GFR). Patients with a 24-hour UPr/e GFR ratio less than 30 were defined as Stage I renal disease, and none of these patients required renal dialysis at 3 years from staging. Patients with the ratio of 30–99, defined as Stage II, had an 11% rate of requiring renal dialysis at 3 years, and among those with Stage III disease, defined as a ratio of 100 or greater, 46% required renal dialysis at 3 years. It must be noted, however, that ABMT has been performed successfully for AL amyloid patients with end-stage renal failure already requiring renal dialysis pre-transplant. This, of course, requires very careful attention to fluid and electrolyte balance, as well as dosing of medications. Batalini and colleagues reported on the Boston Medical Center experience with 32 AL amyloidosis patients with dialysis-dependent end-stage renal failure who underwent autologous hematopoietic transplants between 1994 and 2016 [20].

Compromised hepatic function obviously can impact medication metabolism, and severe liver dysfunction will also increase morbidity risks associated with high-dose therapy. Markers of hepatic function, including prothrombin time, bilirubin level, and transaminases are critical in assessing the degree of liver dysfunction. Although hepatomegaly and splenomegaly are common in AL amyloidosis, severe liver dysfunction due to amyloid is relatively uncommon [21]. However, hypoalbuminemia is common and may be due to either renal involvement by amyloid resulting in proteinuria with loss of albumin in the urine; or hypoalbuminemia may be due to gut malabsorption due to intestinal tract involvement by amyloidosis—as well as the less likely possibility of impaired hepatic synthesis. If gut malabsorption is a significant issue, and ABMT is a consideration, then temporary parenteral nutrition would appear a reasonable means to support a patient until the production of new amyloid can be stopped through antineoplastic therapy.

Pulmonary involvement by AL amyloidosis is a frequent finding but is often clinically silent. When pulmonary amyloidosis does manifest, it most commonly manifests as diffuse alveolar-septal deposition [22]. This can cause ventilation-perfusion mismatch and shunting physiology requiring supplemental oxygen and may improve after ABMT, although the improvement may not manifest until months after transplant.

Gertz from the Mayo Clinic recently published a review of immunoglobulin light chain amyloidosis, in which, he highlighted general criteria for transplant [23]. In his paper, he described patient characteristics associated with a safe outcome—that is, low transplant-related mortality—including systolic blood pressure above 90 mm Hg; troponin level less than 0.06 ng/mL; age below 70 years, and serum creatinine of less than 1.8 mg/dL. For AL amyloid patients who are not deemed transplant candidates, regimens such as conventional-dose melphalan with corticosteroids, the regimen of cyclophosphamide with bortezomib and dexamethasone ("CyBorD"), and the monoclonal antibody daratumumab were suggested. Indeed, early results from the safety run-in portion of the international, multicenter phase III ANDROMEDA study were recently published [24]. In this study, newly diagnosed AL amyloidosis patients are randomized to either CyBorD or CyBorD with subcutaneous daratumumab. Palladini and colleagues reported their outcome data from 28 patients treated in the context of the safety run-in therapy of the arm consisting of CyBorD plus daratumumab, with the daratumumab administered subcutaneously weekly in cycles 1 and 2, then every 2 weeks during cycles 3–6, and then once every 4 weeks for up to 2 years. Patients included in the analysis received a median of 16 treatment cycles at the time of analysis for publication. No grade 5 treatment-related adverse events occurred. Of the 28 patients, 5 died, of whom

3 had proceeded to transplant. The overall hematologic response rate was 96% in this cohort, with a complete hematologic response of 54%. Thus, the approach of CyBorD with daratumumab appears to be a promising bridge to transplant for patients who are deemed not eligible for ABMT as upfront therapy.

Huang and colleagues at Nanjing University performed a prospective, randomized trial comparing induction therapy using two cycles of bortezomib with dexamethasone followed by ABMT, versus ABMT alone. In this study, 56 patients were enrolled, with 28 patients in each arm [25]. With a median follow up of 28 months, the survival at 24 months after the initiation of treatment was 95% in the group that was treated using induction followed by transplant, versus 69.4% survival at 24 months for the group that received transplant without induction. These investigators stated that their preliminary data suggested that the outcome was superior with induction followed by ABMT as compared to ABMT alone. However, data regarding the nature and the role of induction therapy is evolving rapidly with the introduction of newer treatments, and as of this writing, for patients with adequate organ function as delineated by Gertz above, upfront transplant appears to remain an appropriate approach.

A general application of risk stratification to decision-making regarding ABMT for AL amyloidosis has been incorporated into practice guidelines published by the National Cancer Center Network (NCCN), a consortium of cancer centers in the United States that have the designation of Comprehensive Cancer Center from the National Cancer Institute of the United States federal government. Thought leaders from these institutions have, for several decades, been publishing clinical practice guidelines for the management of the relatively common malignancies. In a recent iteration of these guidelines, labeled "NCCN Guidelines Version 1.2021 Systemic Light Chain Amyloidosis," the guidelines use the Revised prognostic staging system for light chain amyloidosis incorporating cardiac biomarkers and serum free light chain measurements, as published by Kumar, Dispenzieri, Lacy, et al., published in the Journal of Clinical Oncology in 2012 **(17, op cit)**. These guidelines recommend primary therapy using the combination of daratumumab—in the subcutaneous form—together with the regimen of cyclophosphamide, bortezomib, and dexamethasone (Dara-CyBorD). This is then followed by ABMT if the patient is deemed appropriate for ABMT. For patients with very small clonal burdens, induction therapy may not be necessary, and ABMT as initial therapy may be the optimal approach (web address: nccnb.org/professionals/physician_gls/pdf/amyloidosis.pdf).

4. Stem cell harvesting

There is a significant body of literature detailing experiences with various approaches to priming for peripheral blood hematopoietic progenitor collection for AL amyloidosis. Due to end-organ damage by the amyloid protein deposition, the morbidity of stem cell collection is significantly higher for patients with AL amyloidosis as compared to patients with multiple myeloma; in one relatively early study, mortality from stem cell collection was as high as 4% of patients [26]. In a recent review paper, Gertz and Schonland summarized nine clinical reports that included analysis of clinical experience with various mobilization approaches [27]. The majority of these reports describe the use of granulocyte-colony stimulating factor (G-CSF) as a single agent (most often 10 mg/kg body weight subcutaneously daily beginning 4–5 days prior to the start of harvesting and continuing until target stem cell collection is obtained, with a goal usually of 5–10 million CD34 cells per kg body weight), with grade 2 or greater toxicities ranging between approximately 4%

and 25%. The most frequent significant toxicity reported is fluid retention, which is attributed to the G-CSF use in the setting of cardiac and/or renal disease. For patients who fail to attain target CD34 cell collection, the protein drug plerixafor—breaks the bond between CXCR-4 and SDF-1 that anchors hematopoietic progenitor cells to the marrow microenvironment—has been used successfully, adding only modestly to reported toxicity. Regimens using chemotherapy agents in addition to recombinant cytokines to stimulate the mobilization of stem cells into the peripheral circulation have been associated with increased morbidity [28].

5. Post-transplant therapy

Investigators at the Ohio State University reported a retrospective analysis of 50 patients with AL amyloidosis who underwent ABMT at that institution. Of this series, 28 patients received post-ABMT maintenance therapy and 22 patients did not. Kaplan–Meier analysis was employed to examine the effect of maintenance versus no maintenance, and found no statistical difference between the groups with respect to either progression-free survival or with respect to overall survival [29]. However, a number of clinical trials have been ongoing to examine the role of post-transplant maintenance therapy. Investigators at Memorial Sloan Kettering Cancer Center have been studying bortezomib with dexamethasone as induction therapy, followed by ABMT, and then followed by maintenance bortezomib with dexamethasone. Preliminary data from this approach has been listed on the Clinical Trials.Gov website for the study. For the 19 patients with AL amyloidosis enrolled, approximately 37% achieved a complete response, with an additional 21% achieving a partial response, and approximately 5% found to have the stable disease; progression of disease was reported in only approximately 5% of patients (clinicaltrials.gov, identifier NCT 01383759). As of this writing, it is too soon to make a definitive statement regarding the role of post-ABMT maintenance therapy, and currently, practices vary between different transplant centers.

6. Future directions

The introduction of new antineoplastic therapies effective in treating plasma cell dyscrasias with novel mechanisms of action, which has occurred over the past two decades—in especial the proteasome inhibitors and more recently monoclonal antibodies—has had a substantial impact on the management approach to multiple myeloma. It is anticipated that just as the landscape has changed for patients with myeloma, changes in the management of patients with systemic AL amyloidosis will follow. However, as is evident from the discussion above, myeloma patients and systemic AL amyloidosis patients are very different clinically, even though they share common biological features. In part because of the relative rarity of systemic AL amyloidosis, and in part because so many patients are diagnosed at a point in time when end-organ dysfunction precludes safe application of ABMT, large, prospective randomized clinical trials will continue to be a challenge for advancing improvements in therapy for this disease. However, much progress has been made in the past quarter-century, and with better recognition of AL amyloidosis and earlier diagnosis, along with new therapeutic modalities, continued improvements in outcome may be anticipated.

Author details

Ivetta Danylesko[1,2]

1 Department of Bone Marrow Transplant, Sheba Medical Center, Ramat Gan, Israel

2 Lecturer, School of Medicine, Tel Aviv University, Tel Aviv, Israel

*Address all correspondence to: alexivetta@gmail.com

References

[1] Blokhin N, Larionov L, Perevodchikova N, et al. Clinical experiences with sarcolysin in neoplasticism diseases. Ann NY Acad Sci. 1958;**68**:1128-1132

[2] Maas RE. A comparison of the effect of prednisone and a placebo in the treatment of multiple myeloma. Cancer Chemotherapy Reports. 1962;**16**:257-259

[3] Kyle RA, Gertz MA, Greipp PR, et al. A trial of three regimens for primary amyloidosis: colchicine alone, melphalan and prednisone, and melphalan, prednisone and colchicine. N England J Med. 1997;**336**:1202-1207

[4] Comenzo RL, Vosburgh E, Simms RW, et al. Dose-intensive melphalan with blood stem cell support for the treatment of AL amyloidosis: One-year follow-up in five patients. Blood. 1996;**88**(1):2801-2806

[5] Moreau P, Leblond V, Bourquelot P, et al. Prognostic factors for survival and response after high-dose therapy and autologous stem cell transplantation in systemic AL amyloidosis: a report on 21 patients. British Journal of Haematology. 1998;**101**:766-769

[6] Jaccard A, Moreau P, Leblond V, et al. High-dose melphalan versus melphalan plus dexamethasone for AL amyloidosis. The New England Journal of Medicine. 2007;**357**:1083-1093

[7] Gertz MA, Comenzo R, Falk RH, et al. Definition of organ involvement and treatment response in immunoglobulin light chain amyloidosis: A consensus opinion from the 10th International Symposium on Amyloid and Amyloidosis. American Journal of Hematology. 2005;**79**:319-325

[8] D'Souza A, Dispenzieri A, Wirk B, et al. Improved outcomes after autologous hematopoietic cell transplantation for light chain amyloidosis: A Center for International Blood and Marrow Transplant Research Study. Journal of Clinical Oncology. 2015;**33**:3741-3749

[9] Tandon N, Muchtar E, Sidana S, et al. Revisiting conditioning dose in newly diagnosed light chain amyloidosis undergoing frontline autologous stem cell transplant: Impact on response and survival. Bone Marrow Transplantation. 2017;**52**:1126-1132

[10] Sanchorawala V, Quillen K, Sloan JM, Andrea NT, Seldin DC. Bortezomib and high-dose melphalan conditioning for stem cell transplantation for AL amyloidosis: A pilot study. Hema. 2011;**96**:1890-1892

[11] Guillaume B, Staetmans N, Jaboul M, et al. Allogenic bone marrow transplantation for AL amyloidosis. Bone Marrow Transplantation. 1997;**20**:907-908

[12] Imamura T, Ogata M, Kohno K, et al. Successful reduced intensity allogeneic stem cell transplantation for systemic AL amyloidosis. Amer J Hematol. 2006;**81**:281-283

[13] Dittrich T, Kimmich C, Hegenbart U, Schonland SO. Prognosis and staging of AL amyloidosis. Acta Hematologica. 2020;**143**:388-399

[14] Dispenzieri A, Lacy MQ, Katzmann JA, et al. Absolute values of immunoglobulin free light chains are prognostic in patients with primary systemic amyloidosis undergoing peripheral blood stem cell transplantation. Blood. 2006;**107**(8): 3378-3383

[15] Warsame R, Kumar SK, Gertz MA, et al. Abnormal FISH in patients with immunoglobulin light chain amyloidosis is a risk factor for cardiac involvement

and for death. Blood Cancer Journal. 2015;**5**:e310

[16] Dispenziedrfi A, Gertz MA, Kyle RA, et al. Serum cardiac troponins and N-terminal pro-brain natriuretic peptide: A staging system for primary systemic amyloidosis. Journal of Clinical Oncology. 2004;**22**:3751-3757

[17] Kumar S, Dispenzieri A, Lacy MQ, et al. Revised prognostic staging system for light chain amyloidosis incorporating cardiac biomarkers and serum free light chain measurements. Journal of Clinical Oncology. 2014; **30**:989-995

[18] Macedo AVS, Schwartzmann PV, Moreno de Gusmao B, et al. Advances in the treatment of cardiac amyloidosis. Current Treatment Options in Oncology. 2020;**23**:36-50

[19] Kastritis E, Gavriatopoulou M, Roussou M, et al. Renal outcomes in patients with AL amyloidosis: Prognostic factors, renal response and the impact of therapy. American Journal of Hematology. 2017;**92**:632-639

[20] Batalini F, Econimo L, Quillen K, et al. High-dose melphalan and stem cell transplantation in patients on dialysis due to immunoglobulin light-chain amyloidosis and Monoclonal Immunoglobulin Deposition Disease. Biology of Blood and Marrow Transplantation. 2018;**24**:127-132

[21] Ebert EC, Nager M. Gastrointestinal manifestations of amyloidosis. The American Journal of Gastroenterology. 2008;**103**:776-787

[22] Khoor A, Colby TV. Amyloidosis of the lung. Archives of Pathology & Laboratory Medicine. 2017;**141**:247-254

[23] Gertz M. Immunoglobulin light chain amyloidosis: 2020 update on diagnosis, prognosis, and treatment. American Journal of Hematology. 2020;**95**:848-860

[24] Paladini G, Kastritis E, Maurer MSA, et al. Daratumumab plus CyBorD for patients with newly diagnosed AL amyloidosis: safety run-in results of ANDROMEDA. Blood. 2020;**136**:71-80

[25] Huang X, Wang Q, Chen W, et al. Induction therapy with bortezomib and dexamethasone followed by autologous stem cell transplantation versus autologous stem cell transplantation alone in the treatment of renal AL amyloidosis: A randomized controlled trial. BMC Medicine. 2014;**12**:2. DOI: 10.1186/1741-7015-12-2

[26] Skinner M, Sanchorawala V, Seldin DC, et al. High-dose melphalan and autologous hematopoietic stem-cell transplantation in patients with AL amyloidosis: An 8-year study. Annals of Internal Medicine. 2004;**140**:85-93

[27] Gertz MA, Schonland S. Stem cell mobilization and autologous transplant for immunoglobulin light-chain amyloidosis. Hematol Oncol Clin N Amer. 2020;**34**:1133-1144

[28] Lisenko K, Wuchter P, Hansberg M, et al. Comparison of different stem cell mobilization regimens in AL amyloidosis patients. Biology of Blood and Marrow Transplantation. 2017;**23**:1870-1878

[29] Ozga M, Zhao Q, Benson D, et al. AL amyloidosis: The effect of maintenance therapy on autologous stem cell transplantation outcomes. Journal of Clinical Medicine. 2020;**23**:3778-3789

Chapter 6

Non-Alzheimers Amyloidoses of the Neurological System: Cerebral Amyloid Angiopathy and Familial Amyloid Polyneuropathy

Gilad A. Muth, Jonathan S. Harrison and Rohan Arora

Abstract

Amyloid deposition plays a significant, albeit overlooked, role in neurologic disorders. Deposition of amyloid proteins in both the central and peripheral nervous systems lead to debilitating, and often deadly, organ dysfunction, including cerebral amyloid angiopathy, familial amyloid neuropathy, and Alzheimer's disease (AD). Alzheimer's disease is discussed in some detail in a separate chapter within this book, and therefore will not be discussed in detail in this chapter. In this chapter, we present the pathological mechanisms, disease manifestations, diagnostic approach, and treatment modalities for diseases of the nervous system caused by amyloid deposition. While significant strides have been made over the years in identifying key underlying pathologic mechanisms, the medical community's understanding of these rare conditions remain limited. The primary goal of this chapter is to provide additional resources and information for clinicians to help identify these disorders early in their course before they cause irreparable damage to their patients.

Keywords: amyloid, neurology, familial amyloid neuropathy, cerebral amyloid neuropathy

1. Introduction

Cerebral amyloid angiopathy (CAA) is a disease of the small and medium vessels of the brain and the leptomeninges. Its hallmark pathological mechanism is the deposition of β-amyloid, a derivation of the amyloid precursor protein (APP), which leads to an array of clinical and radiologic findings. While the prevalence of CAA is challenging to quantify, in an autopsy study from the city of Vantaa, Finland, almost 70% of brain autopsy specimens from individuals aged 85 years or older showed some degree of cerebral amyloid deposition [1]. The most prevalent clinical finding is lobar intracerebral hemorrhage [2], which can be seen on gross specimen (**Figure 1**); other presentations can include transient neurologic symptoms, inflammatory leukoencephalopathy contributing to cognitive impairment, or incidental findings of microbleeds or hemosiderosis on MRI. Interestingly, the hallmark of Alzheimer's disease (AD) is also an abnormal deposition of β-amyloid; however, these two diseases are distinctly different, both in the composition of the amyloid, and in the clinical neurologic manifestations.

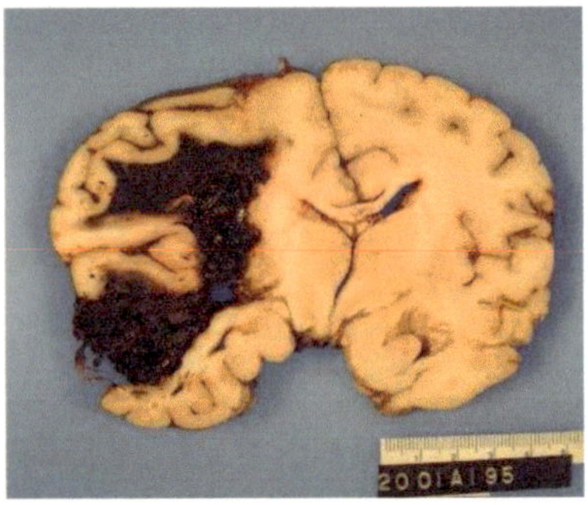

Figure 1.
Lobar intracerebral hemorrhage secondary to amyloid deposition. Photograph courtesy of Roy Rhodes, MD, Professor of Pathology, Louisiana State University Health Sciences Center, New Orleans.

1.1 Pathophysiology

The principal pathologic mechanism that is responsible for CAA is deposition of amyloid protein within the cerebral vasculature; specifically, β-amyloid protein deposition in the tunica media and the adventitia of cortical, subcortical, and leptomeningeal blood vessels. Amyloid can be viewed on histopathologic specimen with Congo Red stain (**Figure 2**). Subsequently, amyloid deposition causes necrosis, focal wall fragmentation and microaneurysms within the vessel walls [3]. These pathologic changes create an environment that leads to subsequent vessel leakage and even frank hemorrhage; these events can recur continuously throughout the course of the disease. The amyloid subtype is classified as β-amyloid, which is derived from the amyloid precursor protein (APP). APP is encoded on human chromosome 21, and is a membrane protein that is highly expressed at neuronal synapses. APP is cleaved by the enzymes beta secratase and gamma secratase to yield Aβ. The Aβ chains may then, in turn, misfold and polymerize, leading to amyloid formation and deposition. The complete mechanism of deposition is not fully understood, however, once deposited, the vasculature is prone to crack [3]. One possible model that has been proposed to promote amyloid deposition is that the mechanism is secondary to impaired clearance of Aβ amyloid through the perivascular drainage pathway [4]. While the APP has been implicated in both CAA and Alzheimer's disease, the subsequent pathology and clinical manifestations diverge quickly based on which isoform of the Aβ amyloid is produced. In CAA, both Aβ 40 and Aβ 42 have been discovered in the walls of the vasculature, however, the Aβ 40 isoform predominates. In AD, Aβ 42 is found in the senile plaques that are histologically pathognomonic for the disease. Researchers also carefully analyzed cerebral

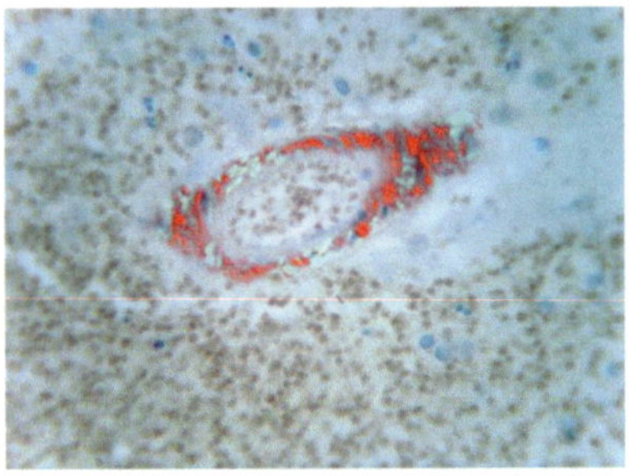

Figure 2.
Amyloid deposition in the cerebral vasculature, visible through Congo Red stain. Photograph courtesy of Roy Rhodes, MD, Professor of Pathology, Louisiana State University Health Sciences Center, New Orleans.

spinal fluid profiles and discovered that samples from CAA and AD patients were decreased in Aβ 40 and Aβ 42 respectively [5].

1.2 Genetics

Overall, CAA is a sporadic disease with no specific driver mutation identified to date; however, genetic susceptibilities have been identified that increase the risk of the disease [6]. Apolipoprotein E (APOE) is a plasma protein that is involved in cholesterol transport, and it exists in three different forms. Abnormalities in the APOE gene, also found to be linked to Alzheimer's disease [7], are seen in some CAA patients; specifically, the e2 or e4 alleles have been found in approximately two thirds of patient with CAA [6]. Furthermore, a dose dependent relationship has been identified for the e2 allele [8]. Patients with the target alleles are at a higher likelihood for CAA related hemorrhage, earlier age of onset of disease, and greater risk for hemorrhage reoccurrence [9]. Ongoing research continues to work to uncover the specific mechanisms and the role of each allele; to date, the understanding is that the e4 allele increases the deposition of the amyloid [10], while the e2 allele changes the integrity of the cerebral vasculature, allowing for cracking and necrosis that predisposes to vessel rupture [10]. The e2 allele is also associated with larger intracerebral hemorrhages, increased mortality, and worse functional outcomes [11].

1.3 Intracerebral hemorrhage

The most prevalent clinical finding associated with CAA is acute intracerebral hemorrhage. Intracerebral hemorrhage secondary to CAA has characteristic imaging features. It is described as a lobar hemorrhage localized to the cortical and subcortical white matter within a hemispheric lobe of the brain (**Figure 3**). This is often compared with hypertensive hemorrhage that is often localized to the deeper structures of the brain, including yet not limited to, the basal ganglia and the putamen [12]. The lobar manifestation often mirrors the underlying distribution of the amyloid deposition, which has been shown to favor cortical vessels. Less commonly, cerebellar or subarachoid/subdural hemorrhage can be found, reflecting involvement of cerebellar or leptomeningeal vasculature [13]. Hemorrhages can occur in any lobe of the cerebrum, however, the lesions are most commonly localized to the posterior regions of the brain. This localization reflects the specific distribution of vascular amyloid deposition, particularly in the vessels of the temporal and occipital lobes [14]. While the direct mechanism and reason is unclear, this is most

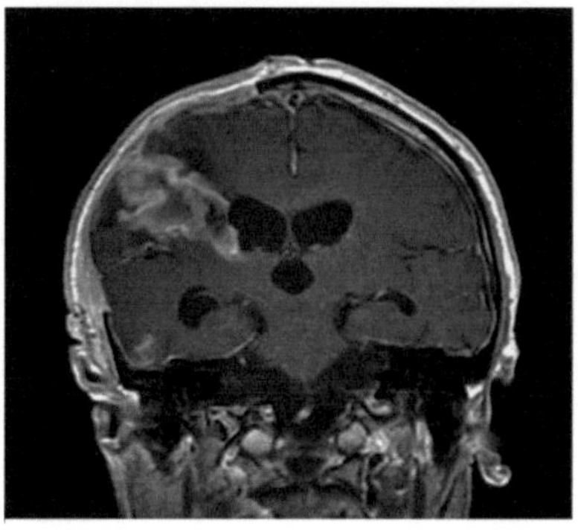

Figure 3.
T1 weighted image demonstrating lobar hemorrhage secondary to amyloid angiopathy. Photograph courtesy of Roy Rhodes, MD, Professor of Pathology, Louisiana State University Health Sciences Center, New Orleans.

likely attributed to differences in tissue composition of the posterior vasculature that allows for easier deposition of amyloid [15]. When amyloid deposition occurs in the leptomeningeal vessels, the hemorrhage can extend beyond brain tissues into the subarachnoid and subdural spaces [16]. It should be noted that gradient-echo or susceptibility weighted sequence brain MRI can reveal cortical microbleeds, and this may be helpful in the diagnosis when identified; these findings are usually asymptomatic and can be found in the juxtacortical and cortical lobar regions, preferring the temporal and occipital lobes.

Similar to the presentation of acute ischemic stroke, the clinical signs and symptoms of intracerebral hemorrhage associated with CAA depend on the location and size of the lesion. Unfortunately, given the wide array of non-specific clinical symptoms, the accurate diagnosis of CAA remains incredibly challenging even for the most adept clinician. Currently, the only definitive diagnostic tool is a brain biopsy, which is rarely performed in vivo and often differed to autopsy. Clinicians can localize the site of the hemorrhage based on clinical presentation. Associated symptoms include headache, seizures, or changes in level of consciousness. The imaging revolution of the late twentieth century was instrumental in the development of the Boston Criteria, a validated set of criteria that has helped clinicians make the diagnosis of CAA using a combination of clinical signs and symptoms, and imaging features, or by pathologic specimen [17]. To date, the Boston Criteria is used as the primary foundation for research and treatment options for CAA; the criteria will be discussed further below.

1.3.1 Diagnosis

While our understanding of the disease process has significantly improved since it was first described, and even more so since imaging technology has evolved, the diagnosis of CAA still remains somewhat elusive. Similar to many other neurologic conditions, a definitive diagnosis can generally only be established post-mortem, based upon pathologic examination. The pathologist can view amyloid deposition on microscopic analysis, as well as see the hemorrhages on macroscopic examination. In clinical practice, clinical suspicion and MRI are the primary tools at the physician's disposal. CAA should be high on the differential diagnosis if MRI findings are positive for lobar hemorrhage without alternative explanation [17]. Advanced age will also support the diagnosis. Brain biopsy can be used; however, it is rarely performed in this setting.

The Boston Criteria, along with its updated modified version, is currently used to diagnose cerebral amyloid angiopathy. A recent paper by Greenberg and colleagues from the Massachusetts General Hospital details the evolution of the Boston Criteria [18]. The Boston Criteria were published initially in the year 1995. The authors stated that the key diagnostic category for the purpose of clinical care and for research is the category of "probable CAA", as this appeared to come closest to defining the disease short of tissue biopsy. In these cases of probable CAA, neuroimaging demonstrates multiple hemorrhages restricted to lobar regions of the brain. A modification to include blood or blood derivatives on imaging, in cortical sulci as one additional hemorrhagic lesion was added to the criteria in the year 2010. This addition is the basis for the "modified Boston Criteria". MRI of the brain is the essential tool for imaging in the Boston Criteria. The Boston Criteria has been validated through multiple studies, comparing it to the gold standards such as pathologic specimens [19].

1.3.2 Prognosis

Prognosis of intracerebral hemorrhage depends on several factors. Bleeds localized superficially will be less likely to cause any mass effects and will not impede on the ventricles. Older patients with larger bleeds have less favorable outcomes. Overall, the mortality associated with intracerebral bleeds ranges from 10 to 30% [20]. Proper management can decrease the likelihood of hemorrhagic recurrence, however, it is not a guarantee. Patients with a prior ICH are 6 times as likely to have another event than those who have never had one [21].

1.4 Microbleeds and superficial siderosis

While intracerebral hemorrhage is the most common clinical and radiologic feature of CAA, there are other radiologic aspects of the disease that are important to mention, including microbleeds and cortical superficial siderosis. Both features are found incidentally on imaging. Microbleeds in the cortical areas are pathognomonic for CAA. They reflect tiny areas of hemosiderin deposition on gradient echo or other T2 weighted sequences that arise from small vessel disease and primarily appear in areas with significant amyloid deposition [22]. See **Figure 4** for a radiographic image of the microbleeds.

The other incidental imaging finding associated with CAA is cortical superficial siderosis (cSS), defined as remote, chronic bleeding in cortical sulci. The finding is usually asymptomatic; however, it is a harbinger for higher risk of intracerebral hemorrhage [23]. It is a common finding in patients with CAA [24] and rarely found in patients with ICH unrelated to CAA [25]; the association ultimately led to the inclusion of cSS in the modified Boston criteria [24]. Unfortunately, it predicts poor functional outcome [26].

1.5 Transient focal neurologic episodes

An associated, albeit rare clinical feature of CAA are transient focal neurologic episodes (TFNE) [27]. These episodes are characterized as recurrent, brief episodes consisting of weakness, numbness, and paresthesias. In addition, patients describe that the symptoms spread over contiguous body parts. Most likely, TFNE represent deficiencies in the activity of cortical areas secondary to small hemorrhages. Given the non-specific nature of the symptomatology, the diagnosis and subsequent management of TFNE remains challenging. Key features that suggest TFNE as opposed to similar transient neurologic conditions such as migraines or seizure are

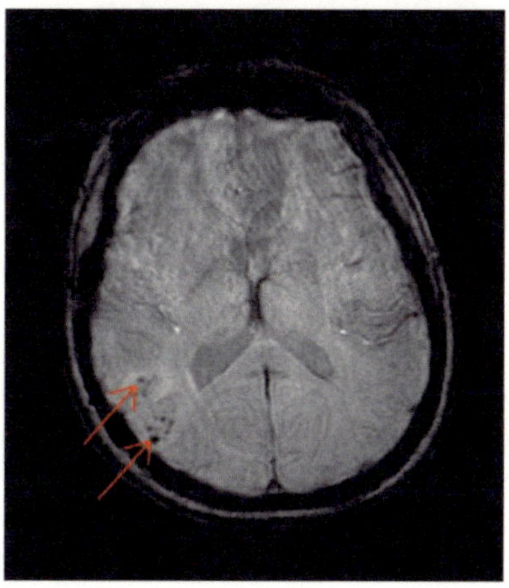

Figure 4.
Axial MRI susceptible weighted imaging of chronic microbleeds in the subcortical white matter of the temporal lobes, in a pattern typical for cerebral amyloid angiopathy. Courtesy of Dr. Shlomo Minkowitz, Assistant Professor of Radiology at Weill Cornell Medicine, New York, NY.

the recurrent nature that is localized to the site of prior lobar hemorrhage. Brain MRI with gradient echo can be used to identify convexity subarachnoid hemorrhage (cSAH), cSS, or CMBs in the cortical regions corresponding to TFNE symptoms. Interestingly, TFNEs are associated with cSS; in one study, CAA patients with TFNE were more likely to have cSS or cSAH than not [28]. In addition, tests to rule out other diagnoses can be considered in order to avoid misdiagnosis and subsequent inappropriate treatment. A case series of CAA patients with TFNE demonstrated that these patients have higher risks of intracerebral hemorrhage [29]. Proper diagnosis can avoid possible mistreatment with tPA for a presumed stroke which can increase the hemorrhagic burden of the disease.

1.6 Cerebral amyloid angiopathy related inflammation and beta-amyloid related angiitis

Cerebral amyloid angiopathy related inflammation (CAA-ri) and beta-amyloid related angiitis (ABRA) are distinct processes, but both are caused by an inflammatory response to Aβ amyloid deposition. Both processes present with a distinct clinical picture that is characterized as subacute and progressive [30]. Symptoms include cognitive decline, mental status changes, seizures, headaches, and focal neurologic deficits [31]. Interestingly, while both processes occur secondary to inflammation, the clinical course of ABRA is typically more insidious, possibly mirroring the findings of histopathologic exam. CAA-ri is associated with perivascular inflammation, while ABRA is described as transmural granulomatous inflammatory infiltrates, similar to what is observed in CNS vasculitis [32]. The rapid evolution of ABRA can lead to herniation if not identified and treated early [33]. While not as common as ICH, CAA-ri manifests earlier than the other findings of CAA [34]. Diagnostic criteria based on clinical and radiographic findings have been developed and validated for CAA-ri [34]. "Probably CAA-ri" is defined as having at least 1 typical clinical feature, asymmetric hyperintensities on T2-weighted MRI, previous evidence of CAA on susceptibility-weighted MRI, and absence of other causes. Definitive diagnosis can only be made on biopsy which would reveal confirmation of perivascular, transmural, or intramural inflammation along with amyloid deposition within the vasculature within the territory normally affected by CAA. These criteria were validated with a sensitivity of 82% and specificity of 97% in a clinical analysis [35]. Other laboratory findings include a normal ESR and CRP [34], and normal CSF analysis with pleocytosis and mildly elevated CSF protein [36]. A case report describes evidence of increased autoantibodies against amyloid in the CSF, pointing to a possible autoimmune response produced by the Aβ deposits [37]. Treatment involves the use of immunosuppression. Typical regimen involves a 5-day course of methylprednisolone followed by an oral steroid taper [38].

1.7 Cognitive impairment

Cognitive impairment has been associated with advanced CAA. In fact, on neuropsychological testing, most CAA patients demonstrate impairments of at least one domain [39]. A clinical-pathological study showed that moderate to severe CAA is associated with faster rates of cognitive decline [40]. The population-based Medical Research Council clinical-pathologic series found a odds ratio for dementia in CAA patients of 7.7 (95% CI, 3.3–20.4) [41]. As mentioned before, Aβ amyloid plays a role in the pathophysiology of Alzheimer's disease, leading researchers to further analyze the connections between the two similar, albeit distinct pathologies. In one autopsy series, CAA was found in 26% of Alzheimer's disease brains [42].

In addition, vascular disease may play a role in cognitive impairment in CAA. Studies demonstrate a correlation between the existence and prevalence of microbleeds and cognitive impairment suggesting that cerebral vascular disease may contribute to clinical neurologic dysfunction [43].

1.8 Management

Once diagnosed, the primary management goal of CAA is focused on prevention of recurrent hemorrhage. As mentioned before, studies revealed that patients with previous hemorrhage are at increased risk of recurrent hemorrhage, and as the number of incident hemorrhages increase, the risk of a subsequent event also increases. A thorough medicine reconciliation is imperative to assess the needs of the patient given any comorbid conditions and medication risks.

1.8.1 Anticoagulation and antiplatelet therapy

The evaluation of anticoagulative and antiplatelet agents is crucial to assess risk of future hemorrhages and needs to be individualized for each patient. Initial assessment of the patient should include factors such as prior intracerebral hemorrhage, presence of other imaging findings, class of antithrombotic agent being used (warfarin, DOACs, ASA, etc.), and the duration of treatment. Patients who are at high risk for thromboembolic events (e.g. cancer patients, patients with underlying hypercoagulable conditions, mechanical heart valves, etc.) might need treatment in order to prevent thrombotic, and subsequent ischemic, events. In addition, atherosclerotic disease and atrial fibrillation need to be managed appropriately in order to decrease risks of thrombosis. New onset ischemic stroke, pulmonary embolism, and myocardial infarction need to be managed with considerable care since intravenous thrombolysis is contraindicated in the setting of intracerebral hemorrhage [44]. In certain cases, endovascular repair and mechanical thrombectomy can be used in lieu of tPA.

1.8.2 Anti-hypertensives

While hypertensive strokes are usually associated with small vessel disease of the inner brain areas, special attention needs to be placed on blood pressure management. The PROGRESS Trial examined the effects of perindopril-based lowering of blood pressure on the evolution of intracerebral hemorrhage (ICH) in the setting of clinically defined CAA [45]. In this multicenter, randomized, placebo-controlled trial, 6105 patients with cerebrovascular disease were assigned to blood pressure reduction using either perindopril, and in some cases together with indapamide, or placebo. Outcomes were assessed as either: probable CAA related ICH as defined by the Boston Criteria, probable hypertension related ICH, and unclassified ICH. With a median follow up of 3.9 years at the time of publication, the authors reported 16 cases of probable CAA-related ICH, 51 probable hypertension related ICH, and 44 unclassified cases of ICH. Active treatment reduced the risk of CAA-related ICH by 77% in this study. The authors concluded that therapy to lower blood pressure is of value in providing some degree of protection against ICH in CAA. A subset analysis of the PROGRESS trial showed that patients with probable CAA and ICH had fewer hemorrhagic recurrences if their blood pressure was tightly controlled on perindopril [46]. Furthermore, an observational cohort study of patients with known ICH continued to have higher risks of recurrent lobar hemorrhage if their blood pressure was inadequately controlled [47].

1.8.3 Statins

The role of statin therapy in the management of CAA and potential or recurrent ICH seems paradoxical given the current understanding of the role of statins in preventing vascular events. The SPARCL trial showed an increased incidence of ICH in the statin arm compared to placebo. Given these results, the trial investigators recommended that perhaps statins should be avoided in patients with a history of ICH [48]. In addition, retrospective analysis of patients with ICH treated with statins showed increased incidence of microbleeds, particularly in cortex and subcortex [49]. Current recommendations are to avoid statins in survivors of ICH [50], however, further investigations revealed that use of statins prior to ICH was associated with reduced mortality and disability at 90 days [51]. In addition, a meta-analysis showed no increase in ICH in patients taking a statin once they developed radiologic evidence of ICH [52].

2. Familial amyloid polyneuropathy

Familial amyloid polyneuropathy (FAP) represents a group of multisystem, life-threatening disorders characterized by the deposition of amyloid protein in either the peripheral motor nervous system, the sensory system, or the autonomic nervous systems, or in a combination of these subsets of the nervous system. These disorders are hereditary forms of amyloidosis, which are typically inherited in an autosomal dominant manner [53]. FAP was first described by Andrade in north Portugal in 1952 [54], and subsequently was described in Japan [55] and Sweden [56]. To date, three main proteins are implicated in the pathogenesis of the majority of cases of FAP: transthyretin, apolipoprotein A-1, and gelsolin. The extent of neurological and non-neurologic organ system involvement is variable, depending on the precursor protein, making the diagnosis often quite challenging. Early and accurate diagnosis is necessary to guide further testing, and subsequent treatment options, and could also contribute to improved research strategies to augment understanding of the pathophysiology and improve therapy.

2.1 ATTR amyloidosis

The most common type of familial amyloid polyneuropathy is caused by the misfolding of transthyretin. Transthyretin, the gene for which is located on human chromosome 18 [57], is produced in the liver, and under normal physiologic conditions, it is responsible for the transport of thyroxin as well as binding of retinol. Due to the electrophoretic mobility of transthyretin, it was originally named prealbumin. While researchers have identified many mutations responsible for the development of amyloid secondary to transthyretin, the substitution for methionine for valine at position 30 of the transthyretin gene is the most common mutation [58]. However, despite the simple missense mutation, disease phenotype is widely variable in severity, symptomatology, and age of onset [59].

2.2 Additional mutations causing FAP

Mutations in the apolipoprotein A1 (APOA1), a protein that is synthesized mainly in the small intestine and liver, is also associated with FAP. It was first described by van Allen in Iowa [60]. While at least 16 mutations have been identified in the APOA1 gene that are associated with amyloidosis [61], neuropathic symptoms are only associated with the Gly26arg mutation [62]. Similar to FAP caused by TTR, APOA1 amyloid also causes a length-dependent polyneuropathy; however, polyneuropathy is not the primary feature of this disease. Renal, hepatic, and gastrointestinal symptoms are the most frequently documented symptoms. Treatment is mainly supportive at present, and is geared toward relief of symptoms. Hepatorenal transplantation for end stage renal disease has been associated with a decrease in concentration of plasma amyloidogenic proteins along with improvement of neuropathic symptoms [63].

Gelsolin-related FAP was first described in Finland in 1969, and it is referred to as the Finish type of amyloidosis [64]. The gelsolin gene is located on chromosome 9, and is a protein that normally binds to actin, and regulates the assembly and disassembly of filaments. Mutations in the gene increase the rate of gelsolin cleavage and cause amyloidosis [65]. Gelsolin amyloid is characterized by the triad of cranial neuropathies, corneal lattice dystrophy, and cutis laxa [66]. Amyloid deposition in gelsolin-related FAP affects the upper branch of the facial nerve, leading to bilateral facial paresis and reduced facial expressions; there is also involvement of the hypoglossal, glossopharyngeal, and vagus nerves. Patients typically begin to complain initially of symptoms of sensory neuropathy around the 5th and 6th decade of life, in a distribution which affects the lower extremeties. In addition, there are reports of autonomic involvement in this variant of FAP [67]. Amyloid deposition can also affect the central nervous system in gelsolin-related FAP; gelsolin amyloid can cause an angiopathy leading to vascular malformations in the brain and spinal cord [68]. To date, no specific treatment has been developed for gelsolin amyloidosis. Management is currently focused on proper ophthalmologic care, and plastic surgery for facial laxity [69].

2.3 Signs and symptoms

One of the key features of FAP that distinguishes it from other neuropathy presentations is that it typically involves multiple areas of the nervous system, with focal neuropathies, sensorimotor polyneuropathies, and autonomic neuropathies. The most recognized manifestation of focal neuropathy is carpal tunnel syndrome, which occurs secondary to endoneurial amyloid deposits of the median nerve [70]. Similar to idiopathic carpal tunnel syndrome, patients usually experience paresthesias in the thumbs and the second and third digits of the hands, along with significant wrist pain. The symptoms experienced with FAP are usually significantly more severe than in idiopathic carpal tunnel syndrome [70]. The sensorimotor neuropathy of FAP is a length dependent neuropathy that affects the small myelinated and unmyelinated fibers first [71]. Patients will initially describe symptoms of foot discomfort, characterized as numbness, paresthesias, and allodynia. On neurologic exam, patients will have decreased pin prick and impaired thermal sensation. With disease onset, light touch, proprioception, motor strength and reflex will be primarily preserved, however, as the disease progresses and affects larger sensory and motor nerve fibers, patients will begin to note deficit changes in these areas as well. Patients will, over time, exhibit significant weakness in their hands and feet, decreased or absent ankle reflexes, and diminished vibration and proprioception in the distal distributions of the nerves. The disease will continue to travel proximally, involving the proximal lower extremities, truck, and the upper extremities. Patients then will begin to have difficulty with ambulation, secondary to their loss of muscle strength and proprioception. Patients will then often start to develop joint deformities (e.g. Charcot joints) as well as plantar ulcers, because of the lack of sensation in their feet [58].

Patients with FAP show significant autonomic dysfunctions as well, particularly with the early age onset form. Typical sequelae of autonomic dysfunction affecting the cardiovascular, genitourinary, and gastrointestinal systems will be present.

Patients will exhibit signs and symptoms of orthostatic hypotension, including light headedness, dizziness, fatigue, and blurry vision upon standing. Patients often develop postprandial diarrhea and/or constipation, as well as post-prandial vomiting due to gastroparesis. In particular, the autonomic control of the cardiovascular, genitourinary, and gastrointestinal systems are affected. With regard to the genitourinary system, symptoms may include urinary retention and incontinence, as well as sexual dysfunction. However, it is important to note that FAP is not associated with central nervous system involvement [58].

2.4 Pathophysiology

The key pathologic step in the development of FAP is the misfolding of the transthyretin protein, which leads to pathologic deposition within the nervous system. Under normal physiologic conditions, TTR is a tetrameric protein with surface receptors that bind retinol and thyroxine, and then carries these in the circulation [72]. TTR is mainly produced in the liver, but also in the retinal pigment epithelium of the eyes and choroid plexus [73]. There are also reports of TTR synthesis in the neurons [74] and peripheral nerve Schwann cells [75]. Upon pathologic misfolding, ATTR deposits unevenly throughout the nervous system. As the ATTR accumulates, it causes pathology through damage to the nerves by mechanical compression, blood vessel invasion, and the toxicity of fibrils to normal cellular and organ structures [58]. Although many mutations have been identified in the TTR gene in patients with ATTR amyloidosis, there are also many cases with so-called wild-type ATTR amyloidosis. In these latter cases, there is abnormal folding of the TTR peptides, but no mutation identified. The molecular pathophysiology in these cases remains to be fully elucidated.

2.5 Diagnosis

The diagnosis of FAP can be elusive, considering the relatively low incidence and the non-specific constellation of symptoms. In fact, the differential diagnosis of polyneuropathy is quite wide (see **Table 1**). As always, a thorough history can potentially help tease out the diagnosis. In endemic areas, a family history can help make the diagnosis more straightforward, when taken together with the constellation of clinical involvement by signs and symptoms. Molecular diagnostics—that is, DNA sequencing, either by rapid allele specific oligonucleotide nucleic acid amplification, or by actual sequencing, will help secure the diagnosis. However, the diagnosis can be quite challenging in patients without a family history of FAP. In sporadic cases, keys to the proper diagnosis include the progressive nature of the disease affecting autonomic, sensory, and motor components of the nervous system, in addition to involvement of other organs affected by amyloid deposition (e.g. cardiac involvement, carpal tunnel syndrome). Since neuropathy is often one of the initial presenting symptoms, it is important that clinicians rule out some of the more common causes of neuropathy first. A useful adjunct to diagnosis, typically done prior to molecular diagnostic studies, is Nerve Conduction Velocity (NCV) studies and electromyography, which will document the specific areas of and electrical features of the neuropathy. Formal autonomic nervous system, including Quantitative Sudomotor Axon Reflex Testing (QSART) will document the extent of dysautonomia. These are typically not specific for FAP, however. Biopsy of a peripheral nerve may demonstrate amyloid, and analysis of the amyloid material in the biopsy by High Performance Liquid Chromatography and Mass Spectroscopy may confirm the amyloid as being composed of ATTR. This is definitive for a diagnosis of FAP, and in such a case, molecular diagnostics are an adjunct that will

Metabolic	Inflammatory
Diabetes End stage renal disease (uremic polyneuropathy) Hypothyroidism Vitamin deficiency (B6, B 12) Chronic liver disease Hypothyroidism Acromegaly Critical illness related	Amyloidosis Monoclonal gammopathy (multiple myeloma, plasmacytoma) Guillain-Barre Chronic idiopathic axonal polyneuropathy Monoclonal gammopathies Connective tissue disease Vasculitis Sarcoidosis Chronic inflammatory demyelinating polyneuropathy Paraneoplastic syndromes Lymphoma
Toxic	**Hereditary**
Alcohol abuse Medication (amiodarone, isoniazid) Chemotherapy Heavy metal exposure Organophosphates Vitamin B6 excess	Charcot-Marie-Tooth Metabolic disorder (Krabbe disease, mitochondrial disorders) Porphyria Familial amyloidosis Sensory/autonomic neuropathies Liability to pressure palsies Metachromic leukodystrophy
Infectious	
HIV infection Lyme disease Syphilis Leprosy West Nile Hepatitis C (cryoglobulinemia)	

Table 1.
Differential diagnosis of familial amyloid polyneuropathy.

allow testing of family members. However, nerve biopsy is invasive, and does carry the risk of causing neurologic damage itself.

2.6 Treatment

The treatment of FAP has progressed significantly over the years since the first cases were reported. The changes in disease therapy are a reflection of developments in the understanding of the disease pathobiology, as well as the advancements in medical treatment overall. The approach to treatment is divided into interventions for symptomatic relief, on the one hand, and disease modifying agents on the other hand. Common anticonvulsants such a gabapentin and pregabalin [76] are used to ameliorate symptoms, as well as antidepressants such as the tricyclic antidepressants (TCAs) [77] and serotonin-norepinephrine reuptake inhibitors (SNRI) [78]. TCAs are particularly helpful in patients who have significant night-time symptoms, given their sedatives properties; however, considerably attention is warranted for exacerbation of autonomic dysfunction. Duloxetine is the most widely used, and studied, SNRI for the treatment of FAP.

2.6.1 Liver transplantation

Liver transplantation has been a treatment option for management of FAP for several decades, based on the understanding that replacing a liver producing defective

TTR with a liver that makes normal TTR protein will improve the long-term outcome. As an example of the results of liver transplantation in this setting, Yamashita and colleagues from Kumamoto University hospital reported on a cohort 80 patients with FAP due to the mutation Val30Met, managed between January 1990 and December 2010. The transplant group consisted of 37 patients who had a partial hepatic graft via living donor transplantation in Japan or who underwent liver transplantation in Sweden, Australia, or the United States. The non-transplant group consisted of 43 patients with FAP. The transplant group had prolonged survival ($p < 0.001$) compared with the non-transplant group. The estimated probability of survival at 10 years was 56.1% for the non-transplant group vs. 100% for the transplant group [79].

2.6.2 Disease modifying agents

The first development in disease modifying agents for FAP occurred with the repurposing of the non-steroidal anti-inflammatory medicine diflusinil. Although liver transplantation has proved to be a successful treatment option, there are many barriers to its use, including availability of technical expertise, availability of a donor, co-morbidities in the patient, and cost. Pre-clinical investigation showed that diflusinil can bind to the thyroxine binding site of the TTR tetramer, and stabilize TTR in the tetramer form, thus preventing the TTR protein subunits from misfolding and being deposited as amyloid. A multicenter, prospective, randomized, double-blind, placebo-controlled clinical trial demonstrated that the use of diflunisal reduces the rate of progression of neurologic impairment [80].

Tafamidis, a thyroxine analogue, is a disease-modifying agent approved for use in the treatment of FAP. Just as diflusinil can stabilize TTR tetramers, it was hypothesized that a synthetic thyroxine analogue may be able to bind to the thyroxin-binding sites on the TTR protein and stabilize the TTR tetramers, similarly preventing them from disassociating, misfolding, and forming amyloid fibrils [81]. A phase III clinical trial in patients with Val30Met ATTR amyloidosis documented delayed progression of neuropathic symptoms with use of Tafamidis, as compared to placebo [82]. An extension study also showed slowing of neuropathy progression [83]. Interestingly, in addition to slowing down the progression of amyloid neuropathy, Tafamidis has also proved effective in improving outcome in ATTR amyloid cardiomyopathy [84].

2.6.3 Gene expression modifying therapy

While stabilization of the TTR tetramer has proved to be somewhat effective in slowing progression of disease, there has, in recent decades, been an active effort to develop genetic modifying therapy in ATTR amyloidosis. Two gene-silencing treatments, Patisiran and Inotersen have been developed and are FDA approved. Patisiran, a small interfering RNA molecule, is delivered parenterally and reduces TTR production [85]. A phase III trial tested Patisiran against placebo; all endpoints were met, including a decrease in neuropathic symptoms and increase in quality of life [86]. Inotersen, an antisense oligonucleotide, was also designed to reduce the production of TTR. A randomized phase III clinical trial in ATTR amyloidosis patients demonstrated a statistically significant decrease in neuropathic impairment [87]. True gene therapy remains to be established for ATTR amyloidosis.

3. Conclusion

Given the constellation of non-specific symptoms, the diagnosis of Cerebral Amyloid Angiopathy and Familial Amyloid Polyneuropathy remains challenging, even to the most adept physician. Despite these challenges, the medical and scientific community's understanding of the diseases has grown considerably since the diseases were first identified and continues to grow, reflected by the increasing number of articles published on the topics. As our knowledge base continues to expand, not only has our ability to make more accurate and timely diagnoses grown stronger, but our treatment and management options have increased as well. It is the authors' hope that the reader has gained a deeper appreciation for the role of amyloid in pathology of the neurologic system and that it will help improve the lives of their patients.

4. Methodology

The information presented in each of the former sections was culled from a literature search using the National Library of Medicine, PubMed website, using key search terms. This involved the search terms amyloidosis, cerebral amyloid angiopathy, and familial amyloid polyneuropathy. From the articles culled, those published in peer reviewed journals were selected for inclusion, most prominently describing initial observations and key clinical trials that advanced therapies.

Author details

Gilad A. Muth[1*], Jonathan S. Harrison[2] and Rohan Arora[3]

1 Prime Health Care Consortium, Denville, New Jersey, USA

2 Rutgers University, Newark, New Jersey, USA

3 Zucker School of Medicine at Hofstra/Northwell, Great Neck, NY, United States

*Address all correspondence to: giladmuth@gmail.com

References

[1] Tanskanen M, Makela M, Myllykangas L, et al. Prevalence and severity of cerebral amyloid angiopathy: A population-based study on very elderly finns (Vantaa 85+). Neuropathology and Applied Neurobiology. 2012;**38**:329-336

[2] Viswanathan A, Greenberg SM. Cerebral amyloid angiopathy in the elderly. Annals of Neurology. 2011;**70**:871-880

[3] Melchor JP, McVoy L, Van Nostrand WE. Charge alterations of E22 enhance the pathogenic properties of the amyloid beta-protein. Journal of Neurochemistry. 2000;**74**:2209-2212

[4] Charidimou A, Gang Q, Werring D. Sporadic cerebral amyloid angiopathy revisited: Recent insights into pathophysiology and clinical spectrum. Journal of Neurology, Neurosurgery & Psychiatry. 2011;**83**:124-137

[5] Charidimou A, Friendrich J, Greenberg S, Viswanathan A. Core cerebrospinal fluid biomarker profile in cerebral amyloid angiopathy. Neurology. 2018;**90**:e754-e762

[6] Nicoll JA, Burnett C, Love S, et al. High frequency of apolipoprotein E epsilon 2 allele in hemorrhage due to cerebral amyloid angiopathy. Annals of Neurology. 1997;**41**:716-721

[7] Schmechel DE, Saunders AM, Strittmatter WJ, et al. Increased amyloid beta-peptide deposition in cerebral cortex as a consequence of apolipoprotein E genotype in late-onset Alzheimer disease. Proceedings of the National Academy of Sciences of the United States of America. 1993;**90**:9649-9653

[8] Rannikmäe K, Samarasekera N, Martînez-Gonzâlez NA, et al. Genetics of cerebral amyloid angiopathy: Systematic review and meta-analysis. Journal of Neurology, Neurosurgery, and Psychiatry. 2013;**84**:901-908

[9] O'Donnell HC, Rosand J, Knudsen KA, et al. Apolipoprotein E genotype and the risk of recurrent lobar intracerebral hemorrhage. The New England Journal of Medicine. 2000;**342**:240-245

[10] Greenberg SM, Vonsattel JP, Segal AZ, et al. Association of apolipoprotein E epsilon 2 and vasculopathy in cerebral amyloid angiopathy. Neurology. 1998;**50**:961-965

[11] Biffi A, Anderson CD, Jagiella JM, et al. APOE genotype and extent of bleeding and outcome in lobar intracerebral haemorrhage: A genetic association study. Lancet Neurology. 2011;**10**:702-709

[12] Park JH, Seo SW, Kim C, et al. Pathogenesis of cerebral microbleeds: In vivo imaging of amyloid and subcortical ischemic small vessel disease in 226 individuals with cognitive impairment. Annals of Neurology. 2013;**73**:584-593

[13] Cuny E, Loiseau H, Castel JP, et al. Amyloid angiopathy-related cerebellar hemorrhage. Surgical Neurology. 1996;**46**:235-239

[14] Rosand J, Smithh EE, Greenberg SM, et al. Spatial clustering of hemorrhages in probable cerebral amyloid angiopathy. Annals of Neurology. 2005;**58**:459-462

[15] Weller RO, Nicoll JA. Cerebral amyloid angiopathy: Both viper and maggot in the brain. Annals of Neurology. 2005;**58**:348-350

[16] Samarasekera N, Rodrigues MA, Toh PS, Salman RA. Imaging features of intracerebral hemorrhage with cerebral amyloid angiopathy: Systematic review and meta-analysis. PLoS One. 2017;**12**

[17] Greenberg SM. Cerebral amyloid angiopathy: Prospects for clinical diagnosis and treatment. Neurology. 1998;**51**:690-694

[18] Greenberg SM, Charidimou A. Diagnosis of cerebral amyloid angiopathy: Evolution of the Boston criteria. Stroke. 2018;**49**:491-497

[19] Knudsen KA, Rosand J, Greenberg SM, Karluk D. Clinical diagnosis of cerebral amyloid angiopathy: Validation of the Boston criteria. Neurology. 2001;**56**:537-539

[20] Kase CS, Williams JP, Wyatt DA, Mohr JP. Lobar intracerebral hematomas: Clinical and CT analysis of 22 cases. Neurology. 1982;**32**:1146-1150

[21] Biffi A, Halpin A, Towfighi A, et al. Aspirin and recurrent intracerebral hemorrhage in cerebral amyloid angiopathy. Neurology. 2010;**75**:693-698

[22] Greenberg SM, Nandigam RN, Delgado P, et al. Microbleeds versus macrobleeds: Evidence for distinct entities. Stroke. 2009;**40**:2382-2386

[23] Charidimou A, Peeters AP, Jäger R, et al. Cortical superficial siderosis and intracerebral hemorrhage risk in cerebral amyloid angiopathy. Neurology. 2013;**81**:1666-1673

[24] Linn J, Halpin A, Demaerel P, et al. Prevalence of superficial siderosis in patients with cerebral amyloid angiopathy. Neurology. 2010;**74**:1346-1350

[25] Charidimou A, Jäger RH, Fox Z, et al. Prevalence and mechanisms of cortical superficial siderosis in cerebral amyloid angiopathy. Neurology. 2013;**81**: 626-632

[26] Wollenweber FA, Opherk C, Zedde M, et al. Prognostic relevance of cortical superficial siderosis in cerebral amyloid angiopathy. Neurology. 2019;**92**:e792-e801

[27] Charidimou A. Cerebral amyloid angiopathy-related transient focal neurological episodes (CAA-TFNEs): A well-defined clinical-radiological syndrome. Journal of the Neurological Sciences. 2019;**406**:116496

[28] Charidimou A, Linn J, Vernooij MW, et al. Cortical superficial siderosis: Detection and clinical significance in cerebral amyloid angiopathy and related conditions. Brain. 2005;**138**:2126-2139

[29] Charidimou A, Peeters A, Fox Z, et al. Spectrum of transient focal neurological episodes in cerebral amyloid angiopathy. Stroke. 2012;**43**: 2324-2330

[30] Eng JA, Frosch MP, Choi K, et al. Clinical manifestations of cerebral amyloid angiopathy related inflammation. Annals of Neurology. 2004;**55**:250-256

[31] Scolding NJ, Joseph F, Kirby PA, et al. Abeta-related angiitis: Primary angiitis of the central nervous system associated with cerebral amyloid angiopathy. Brain. 2005;**128**:500-515

[32] Salvarani C, Hunder GG, Morris JM, et al. AB-related angiitis: Comparison with CAA without inflammation and primary CNS vasculitis. Neurology. 2013;**81**:1596-1603

[33] Ng DW, Magaki S, Terashima KH, et al. Amyloid-β-related angiitis: A report of 2 cases with unusual presentations. Human Pathology. 2017;**64**:191-197

[34] Chung KK, Anderson NE, Hutchinson D, et al. Cerebral amyloid angiopathy related inflammation: Three case reports and a review. Journal of Neurology, Neurosurgery, and Psychiatry. 2001;**82**:20-26

[35] Auriel E, Charidimou A, Edip M, et al. Validation of clinicoradiological criteria

for the diagnosis of cerebral amyloid angiopathy-related inflammation. JAMA Neurology. 2016;**73**:197-202

[36] Hermann DM, Keyvani K, van de Nes J, et al. Brain reactive b-amyloid antibodies in primary CNS angiitis with cerebral amyloid angiopathy. Neurology. 2011;**77**:503-505

[37] DiFrancesco JC, Brioschi M, Brighina L, et al. Anti-Ab autoantibodies in the CSF of a patient with CAA-related inflammation: A case report. Neurology. 2011;**76**:842-844

[38] Reynolds A, Byrd E, Mossa-Basha M, et al. A 61-year-old woman with headaches and aphasia. Neurohospitalist. 2015;**5**:245-250

[39] Greenberg SM, Bacskai BJ, Hernandez-Guillamon M, et al. Cerebral amyloid angiopathy and Alzheimer disease—One peptide, two pathways. Nature Reviews. Neurology. 2020;**16**:30-42

[40] Boyle PA, Yu L, Nag S, et al. Cerebral amyloid angiopathy and cognitive outcomes in community-based older persons. Neurology. 2015;**85**: 1930-1936

[41] Neuropathology Group of the Medical Research Council Cognitive Function and Ageing Study (MRC CFAS). Pathological correlates of late-onset dementia in a multicentre, community-based population in England and Wales. Lancet. 2011;**357**:169-175

[42] Ellis RJ, Olichney JM, Thal LJ, et al. Cerebral amyloid angiopathy in the brains of patients with Alzheimer's disease: The CERAD experience, part XV. Neurology. 1996;**46**:1592-1596

[43] Poels MM, Ikram MA, van der Lugt A, et al. Cerebral microbleeds are associated with worse cognitive function: The Rotterdam Scan Study. Neurology. 2012;**78**:326-333

[44] Powers WJ, Rabinstein AA, Ackerson T, et al. Guidelines for the early management of patients with acute ischemic stroke: 2019 update to the 2018 guidelines for the early management of acute ischemic stroke: A guideline for healthcare professionals from the American Heart Association/American Stroke Association. Stroke. 2019;**50**: e344-e418

[45] Fransen M, Anderson C, Chalmers J, et al. Effects of a perindopril-based blood pressure-lowering regimen on disability and dependency in 6105 patients with cerebrovascular disease. Stroke. 2003;**34**:2333-2338

[46] Arima H, Tzourio C, Anderson C, et al. Effects of perindopril-based lowering of blood pressure on intracerebral hemorrhage related to amyloid angiopathy: The PROGRESS trial. Stroke. 2010;**41**:394-396

[47] Biffi A, Anderson CD, Battey TWK, et al. Association between blood pressure control and risk of recurrent intracerebral hemorrhage. JAMA. 2015;**314**:904-912

[48] Amarenco P, Bogousslavsky J, Callahan A III, et al. Stroke prevention by aggressive reduction in cholesterol levels (SPARCL) investigators. High-dose atorvastatin after stroke or transient ischemic attack. The New England Journal of Medicine. 2006;**355**:549-559

[49] Shoamanesh A, Kwok CS, Lim PA, et al. Postthrombolysis intracranial hemorrhage risk of cerebral microbleeds in acute stroke patients: A systematic review and meta-analysis. International Journal of Stroke. 2012;**8**:348-356

[50] Westover MB, Bianchi MT, Eckman MH, et al. Statin use following intracerebral hemorrhage. Archives of Neurology. 2011;**68**:573-579

[51] Biffi A, Devan WJ, Anderson CD, et al. Statin use and outcome after

intracerebral hemorrhage. Neurology. 2011;**76**:1581-1588

[52] McKinney JS, Kostis WJ. Statin therapy and the risk of intracerebral hemorrhage: A meta-analysis of 31 randomized controlled trials. Stroke. 2012;**43**:2149-2156

[53] Benson M, Kincaid J. The molecular biology and clinical features of amyloid neuropathy. Muscle & Nerve. 2007;**36**: 411-423

[54] Andrade C. A peculiar form of peripheral neuropathy Familial atypical generalized amyloidosis with special involvement of the peripheral nerves. Brain. 1952;**75**:408-427

[55] Araki S, Mawatari S, Ohta M, et al. Polyneuritic amyloidosis in a Japanese family. Archives of Neurology. 1968;**18**:593-602

[56] Andersson R. Familial amyloidosis with polyneuropathy. A clinical study based on patients living in northern Sweden. Acta Medica Scandinavica. 1976;**590**:1-64

[57] Wallace MR, Naylor SL, Kluve-Beckerman B, et al. Localization of the human prealbumin gene to chromosome 18. Biochemical and Biophysical Research Communications. 1985;**129**:753-758

[58] Plante-Bordeneuve V, Said G. Familial amyloid polyneuropathy. Lancet Neurology. 2011;**10**:1086-1097

[59] Planté-Bordeneuve V, Carayol J, Ferreira A, et al. Genetic study of transthyretin amyloid neuropathies: Carrier risks among French and Portuguese families. Journal of Medical Genetics. 2003;**40**:e120

[60] van Allen MW, Frohlich JA, Davis JR. Inherited predisposition to generalized amyloidosis. Clinical and pathological study of a family with neuropathy, nephropathy, and peptic ulcer. Neurology. 1969;**19**:10-25

[61] Eriksson M, Schönland S, Yumlu S, et al. Hereditary apolipoprotein AI-associated amyloidosis in surgical pathology specimens: Identification of three novel mutations in the *APOA1* gene. The Journal of Molecular Diagnostics. 2009;**11**:257-262

[62] Nichols WC, Gregg RE, Brewer HB Jr, et al. A mutation in apolipoprotein A-I in the Iowa type of familial amyloidotic polyneuropathy. Genomics. 1990;**8**:318-323

[63] Testro AG, Brennan SO, Macdonell RA, et al. Hereditary amyloidosis with progressive peripheral neuropathy associated with apolipoprotein AI Gly26Arg: Outcome of hepatorenal transplantation. Liver Transplantation. 2007;**13**:1028-1031

[64] Meretoja J. Familial systemic paramyloidosis with lattice dystrophy of the cornea, progressive cranial neuropathy, skin changes and various internal symptoms: A previously unrecognized heritable syndrome. Annals of Clinical Research. 1969;**1**:314-324

[65] Levy E, Haltia M, Fernandez-Madrid I, et al. Mutation in gelsolin gene in Finnish hereditary amyloidosis. The Journal of Experimental Medicine. 1990;**172**:1865-1867

[66] Kiuru S. Review: Gelsolin-related familial amyloidosis, Finnish type (FAF), and its variants found worldwide. Amyloid. 1998;**5**:55-66

[67] Kiuru S, Seppäläinen AM. Neuropathy in familial amyloidosis, Finnish type (FAF): Electrophysiological studies. Muscle & Nerve. 1994;**17**:299-304

[68] Kiuru S, Salonen O, Haltia M. Gelsolin-related spinal and cerebral amyloid angiopathy. Annals of Neurology. 1999;**45**:305-311

[69] Pihlamaa T, Rautio J, Kiuru-Enari S, et al. Gelsolin amyloidosis as a cause of early aging and progressive bilateral facial paralysis. Plastic and Reconstructive Surgery. 2011;**127**:234-251

[70] Koike H, Morozumi S, Kawagashira Y, et al. The significance of carpal tunnel syndrome in transthyretin Val30Met familial amyloid polyneuropathy. Amyloid. 2009;**16**:142-148

[71] Said G, Ropert A, Faux N. Length dependent degeneration of fibres in Portuguese amyloid polyneuropathy. A clinicopathological study. Neurology. 1984;**34**:1025-1032

[72] Monaco HL, Rizzi M, Coda A. Structure of a complex of two plasma proteins: Transthyretin and retinol-binding protein. Science. 1995;**268**: 1039-1041

[73] Soprano DR, Herbert J, Soprano KJ, et al. Demonstration of transthyretin mRNA in the brain and other extrahepatic tissues in the rat. Journal of Biological Chemistry. 1985;**260**: 11793-11798

[74] Li X, Masliah E, Reixach N, Buxbaum JN. Neuronal production of transthyretin in uman and murine Alzheimer's disease: Is it protective? The Journal of Neuroscience. 2011;**31**: 12483-12490

[75] Murakami T, Ohsawa Y, Zhenghua L, et al. The transthyretin gene is expressed in Schwann cells of peripheral nerves. Brain Research. 2010;**1348**:222-225

[76] Lesser H, Sharma U, LaMoreaux L, Poole RM. Pregabalin relieves symptoms of painful diabetic neuropathy: A randomized controlled trial. Neurology. 2004;**63**:2104-2110

[77] Shlay JC, Chaloner K, Max MB, et al. Acupuncture and amitriptyline for pain due to HIV-related peripheral neuropathy: A randomized controlled trial. Terry Beirn community programs for clinical research on AIDS. JAMA. 1998;**280**:1590-1595

[78] Raskin J, Pritchett YL, Wang F, et al. A double-blind, randomized multicenter trial comparing duloxetine with placebo in the management of diabetic peripheral neuropathic pain. Pain Medicine. 2005;**6**:346-356

[79] Yamashita T, Ando Y, Okamoto S, et al. Long-term survival after liver transplantation in patients with familial amyloid polyneuropathy. Neurology. 2012;**78**:637-643

[80] Berk JL, Suhr OB, Obici L, et al. Repurposing diflunisal for familal amyloid polyneuropathy. JAMA. 2013;**310**:2658-2667

[81] Obici L, Adams D. Acquired and inherited amyloidosis: Knowledge driving patients' care. Journal of the Peripheral Nervous System. 2020;**25**:85-101

[82] Coelho T, Da Silva AM, Maia LF, et al. Tafamidis for transthyretin familial amyloid polyneuropathy: A randomized, controlled trial. Neurology. 2012;**79**:785-792

[83] Barroso FA, Judge DP, Ebede B, et al. Long-term safety and efficacy of tafamidis for the treatment of hereditary transthyretin amyloid polyneuropathy: Results up to 6 years. Amyloid. 2017;**24**:194-204

[84] Maurer MS, Siltan MB, Rapezzi C. Tafamidis for transthyretin amyloid cardiomyopathy. New England Journal of Medicine. 2019;**380**:196-197

[85] Adams D, Koike H, Slama M, Coelho T. Hereditary transthyretin amyloidosis: A model of medical progress for a fatal disease. Nature Reviews Neurology. 2019;**15**:387-404

[86] Adams D, Attarian S, Plante-Bordeneuve V, et al. Patisiran, an

RNAi therapeutic, for hereditary transthyretin amyloidosis. New England Journal of Medicine. 2018;**379**:11-21

[87] Benson MD, Waddington-Cruz M, Berk JL, et al. Inotersen treatment for patients with hereditary transthyretin amyloidosis. The New England Journal of Medicine. 2018;**379**:22-31